Praise for *Damaged*

"I have been pining for this book and Maunder and Hunter did not disappoint. *Damaged* is about a wounded soul whose story you must keep reading. Maunder and Hunter find the love in a patient that many of our colleagues would label 'difficult.' They connect the dots that link strength and vulnerability and those that join the psychological to the physical. With skill and humility, they tell a story about every one of us."
Dr. Brian Goldman, emergency physician, host of CBC's *White Coat, Black Art*, and author of *The Power of Kindness: Why Empathy is Essential in Everyday Life*

"This book is dynamite! *Damaged* is a bold and profoundly important story of two doctors and of one man's monumental struggle. You will find yourself and your family, friends, and co-workers in this phenomenal read. So often the health care system fails the most vulnerable people when it comes to mental health. Maunder and Hunter show not only how the system fails, but the revolution it will take to not just improve, but reengineer a structure of care that truly helps people heal. The vividly clear connection between early childhood trauma and adult physical and mental health issues is an education we all need. This story is a powerful example of what's possible. You will see that we can all contribute, and demand the revolution needed to make things better for everyone."
Clara Hughes, OC, OM, six-time Olympic medalist, and founding spokesperson for Bell Let's Talk

"This narrative is the best teaching tool that I've ever read. The story of Isaac and his therapist, Bob, is more than a model demonstrating the intensity and challenge of providing psychotherapy. The account is humane and transparent and owns the errors in establishing the bonds of trust that enable Isaac to heal over time. It also recounts the remarkable thirty-year relationship of mutual support and reflection shared by two psychiatrists, and of the trials and joys they experience with their patients. The authors

appeal for societal activism on issues of racism, poverty, trauma-based therapy, accessibility, and accountability – the myriad of social injustices that we all tolerate. This is their call for a revolution in care."
Dr. Jean Marmoreo, author and advocate for elders, end-of-life, and medical assistance in dying

Robert Maunder, MD
and Jonathan Hunter, MD

DAMAGED

Childhood Trauma,
Adult Illness, and
the Need for a
Health Care
Revolution

ÆVO UTP

Aevo UTP
An imprint of University of Toronto Press
Toronto Buffalo London
utorontopress.com
© University of Toronto Press 2021

ISBN 978-1-4875-2834-8 (cloth)
ISBN 978-1-4875-2837-9 (EPUB)
ISBN 978-1-4875-2836-2 (PDF)

Library and Archives Canada Cataloguing in Publication

Title: Damaged : childhood trauma, adult illness, and the need for a health care
    revolution / Robert Maunder, MD, and Jonathan Hunter, MD.
Names: Maunder, Bob (Bob G.), author. | Hunter, Jon, 1958– author.
Description: Includes bibliographical references and index.
Identifiers: Canadiana (print) 20210206772 | Canadiana (ebook) 2021020687X |
    ISBN 9781487528348 (cloth) | ISBN 9781487528379 (EPUB) |
    ISBN 9781487528362 (PDF)
Subjects: LCSH: Psychotherapist and patient. | LCSH: Adult child abuse victims –
    Mental health. | LCSH: Child abuse – Psychological aspects. | LCSH: Psychic
    trauma.
Classification: LCC RC480.8 .M38 2021 | DDC 616.89/14–dc23

Printed in Canada

We acknowledge the financial support of the Government of Canada, the
Canada Council for the Arts, and the Ontario Arts Council, an agency of the
Government of Ontario, for our publishing activities.

Canada Council **Conseil des Arts**
for the Arts **du Canada**

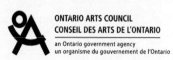

ONTARIO ARTS COUNCIL
CONSEIL DES ARTS DE L'ONTARIO
an Ontario government agency
un organisme du gouvernement de l'Ontario

Funded by the   Financé par le
Government   gouvernement
of Canada   du Canada

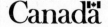

I have spread my dreams under your feet;
Tread softly because you tread on my dreams.
W.B. Yeats

To all the people who raised me, as a child and as an adult,
with grace, security, and love.
Jon

For my parents, my children, and Lynn, who have kept me whole.
Bob

Contents

Preface

Isaac's experiences of childhood abuse twist and stretch his body and his mind like a worm on a hook, even now, well into middle age. This is his story, as told by his psychiatrist of twenty years. They have worked together so closely that Isaac's psychiatrist has lost his objectivity and distance. To be true to Isaac's story, he must reveal himself and how their work has changed him. Indeed, the story of Isaac and his psychiatrist, Bob, is a story of relationships. About how deeply people can affect each other for better and for worse – including people who are ill and the professionals who care for them.

It is also the story of the relationship between two psychiatrists, Bob and Jon – us. We have been friends and collaborators for more than thirty years. Jon specializes in providing psychiatric care for people with cancer, often young adults with bone cancer and women with breast cancer. We are about the same age and share tastes in music and in jokes. We don't make eye contact at funerals because we make each other laugh. We have taught together and worked together on the same projects for so long that people often confuse us. Neither knows who is responsible for our best ideas. The safety and honesty of our relationship helps us both be better doctors and sustains us in the face of relentless vicarious exposure to our patients' traumas.

With Isaac as an example, we have written this book to start a revolution. No kidding. People whose early experiences have caused lifelong damage need a revolution of relationships, specifically a revolution of health care relationships. Millions of adults who share Isaac's experience of disease and suffering caused by early adversity need a health care system that responds to their reality. The changes in health care relationships they need are also revolutionary – doctors and other health care professionals who see and understand their experience, conversations in which they have a voice, and safety from repeated harm.

Of course, Isaac has consented to his story being told and at times urged Bob to tell it. Nonetheless, he has been harmed in the past when others learned about his abuse. We have changed much to protect his anonymity. We are also mindful of our readers. Reading about Isaac's experiences will cause uneasy feelings. We have left out details that were not required to make our points; it is not our intent to shock. But the story of what matters in Isaac's childhood cannot be told without relating some of the particulars. For those who have lived a life that is free of the kinds of experience that Isaac has had, revolution requires unease. But for those who know similar experiences all too well, descriptions can be triggering.

Isaac's experience has much to teach us. If you have not had his experiences, you know someone who has. Childhood adversity that is severe enough to be harmful throughout life affects over sixty million American adults and about nine million Canadian adults. It is one of the biggest public health issues of our time, and yet health care systems are ill-equipped to even acknowledge the problem. Everyone looks away, but looking away makes things worse.

We can learn from Bob's experience as well. It is rare to be allowed into a therapist's office to see and hear what happens there. We have opened the window as wide as we can for you. If you are a psychotherapist or in therapy yourself, a "therapist's eye view" on a very challenging relationship may give you something new to work with. If you are managing on your own the kind of pain that Isaac has endured, we hope Isaac's story will demonstrate how it can help to share that burden.

Stories of childhood abuse tend to resolve into simple narratives: villains and victims, good parents and bad ones, good doctors and bad ones, us and them. If we are going to change the world, everyone needs to realize that there is only us. Real stories are messy; we need you to see the whole mess.

A note about *we* and *I*. We realized in the writing that the narrator of the story could only be Bob, and so it is told in the first-person singular. A switch to *we* when we reflect on the meaning and implications of that story was distracting. So, although we have collaborated equally on all parts of the book, we have told it from Bob's perspective. Jon makes appearances throughout the book as its third main character.

1

"The damage that I am"

Five years ago, Isaac wrote to me to describe the awful sexual abuse he had experienced as a child much more clearly than he had ever managed to say out loud over fifteen years of therapy. Two hours after the next session, in which we discussed the abuse again, I received another email.

> Hi Bob, I was alone again, thinking in the car how much I've had to inflict upon you over the years, perhaps now more than ever. I was also thinking that in the context of what we do, writing is an act of cowardice. Can't say it, so write it.
>
> It's the best I can do right now. For the record, you can do what you want with whatever I write. I want you to save what I've written. Not for me but for you. You can share what I've told you as long as I remain anonymous. Perhaps it will be good for both of us.
>
> I've always asked you for everything you have, no half measures, and once again, I need you to help me understand the damage that I am.

I am Isaac's psychiatrist. He has been driving to my office in a downtown hospital every week or two for twenty years. We're both in our sixties now. If you add up those hours, I have spent more time talking with Isaac than I have with most of my friends, and after twenty years, we're still not done.

I am a doctor who specializes in treating people who have physical and mental issues. My dialogue with Isaac hasn't healed him, emotionally or physically, but it has helped. Both of us are changed. That sums up my experience as a psychiatrist for physically ill people when trying to fix the damage done by childhood trauma. Our work together helps, but it rarely heals, and I am not the person I used to be – better in some ways, I suppose, but also a little bit broken, far humbler about my expertise, and utterly pissed off.

Why? Because there are far too many people like Isaac who suffer the effects of childhood abuse and neglect: about one in three adults, if we are talking about the more severe sorts of abuse. That's about nine million Canadians and over sixty million Americans. Too often, this early traumatic experience makes people sick with serious physical diseases. Beyond that, it is harder than usual for these people to get better. The effects of trauma mess with people's ability to receive good care because health care takes place in relationships, and their relationships are fraught.

Worse: even though Isaac's kind of trouble is common, it is not even part of the medical conversation. Medicine, which has succeeded spectacularly in understanding the biology of disease through increasingly narrow areas of specialization, fails equally spectacularly when it comes to understanding the needs of the whole person, which must include both the mental and the emotional parts. This medical conversation is even more deficient when it comes to understanding the importance of a patient's personal relationships – the main way in which people help and harm each other.

I know the doctors that Isaac has seen; they're good ones, experts. But most have found him difficult to treat – he is too angry, too mistrustful, and too hard to believe. It screws up their craft. A classic paper that called such patients "hateful" appeared in *The New England Journal of Medicine* in 1978 and sorted them into types: dependent clingers, entitled demanders, manipulative help-rejecters, and self-destructive deniers. It would be hard to find language more pejorative or clearer in communicating the worst version of the physician's perspective on seemingly doomed medical relationships.

Doctors see the trouble but don't look for the cause. And they aren't alone. We live in a culture that is complicit in this denial. Frederick Douglass – a former slave who became a US statesman and social reformer – has been credited with saying, "It is easier to build strong children than to repair broken men." Both Isaac and I know, after decades of trying, how hard it is to repair a broken adult. Yet building strong children will not be easier if we look away from abuse. ACE

The idea of ACEs helps us to avoid looking away. It comes from a questionnaire that Vincent Felitti and his colleagues developed in the 1990s to measure childhood adversity. Their work, the adverse childhood experience (ACE) study, scored harmful experiences based on the presence or absence of ten kinds of abuse, neglect, and family troubles. Everyone has an ACE score between zero and ten, with one point allotted for each of those ten types of experiences while growing up. Most people have an ACE score higher than zero, which helps to reduce the "us versus them" tension that leads people to avoid paying attention to childhood adversity.

This early life adversity occurs everywhere – in rich families and in poor, in all cultures, among the uneducated and the elite. Felitti's original ACE study was conducted among the privileged members of a large San Diego health maintenance organization. Eighty per cent of the participants were white and 75 per cent were college educated. We replicated their findings in the family medicine unit at our hospital, also with highly educated patients, most of whom were white. Our similar findings clearly indicate that privilege does not make children immune from adversity. It's our problem – all of us – not just a problem for "them," whoever they are.

While not everyone with ACEs gets sick, the higher your ACE score, the harder it is to avoid the consequences. Many of the negative mental consequences of ACEs are obvious: anxiety disorders, depression, and premature death, including by suicide. This is much of psychiatrists' and other mental health professionals' daily work: helping people who suffer from these disorders to explore the experiences that caused the trouble. Much of the physical risk of ACEs comes from the way people try to cope with this distress. Those with higher ACE scores are more likely to smoke, to drink excessively, to have a child as a teenager, to get a sexually transmitted infection, and to eat to manage their emotions instead of for nutrition. The US Department of Health and Human Services once estimated that ACEs account for somewhere between one-quarter and one-half of the risk for many potentially fatal chronic diseases, such as diseases of the heart, liver, and respiratory system. Shockingly, childhood adversity is a main contributor to the diseases that use up the lion's share of our health care budgets. Given the cascade of negatives that ACEs trigger, they can fairly be called the unacknowledged "cause of causes."

This is why I am telling Isaac's story. Though every person's history is unique, I'm not writing about Isaac because he is special. His story is extreme, but although he is special to me, his story is common; that is the point. I am writing about Isaac because too many of his harrowing experiences are typical and should have been prevented. Isaac has a chronic disease. He has smoked and used prescription and street drugs for most of his life. He is hard to help because he doesn't trust easily, and he is fiercely determined to hide the fear and shame of his childhood experiences, which makes him prickly and intimidating. I am not the only doctor who has called him the most difficult patient they have ever treated.

What I have learned from treating people like Isaac is that our health care systems often go wrong when dealing with adults who are sick because of trauma. Instead of supporting our patients' strengths and helping them to recover, we contribute to their damage. By explicitly identifying circumstances in which our system increases health risks when it could be helping instead, I hope we can open windows of opportunity for change.

Which brings us to revolution through relationship. One meaning of *revolution* is "upheaval." My relationship with Isaac, and others like him, has turned parts of my world upside down. Where I once saw innocence and expected things to be okay, I often now see malign forces and expect harm. Instead of sleeping undisturbed, as I used to, I startle and wake in apprehension. Isaac tells me that our relationship has also upended his world, but for the better. We'll spend much of the rest of the book understanding how that could be when our relationship has provided him with neither cure nor healing.

My relationship with Jon is revolutionary too. I don't know of others in our field who function so closely as a team, more like twins than colleagues or friends sometimes, or who egg each other on, support each other, and co-create the way we have done. We have come to realize that relationships are central to health and to health care. It is within *our* relationship, while puzzling with each other about the relationships that we each have with patients, that we have learned together that health does not occur just within an individual. Health happens between people.

Most of all, *revolution* refers to overthrowing the established social order. Jon and I want to ignite a revolution of awareness of the effects of childhood trauma on lifelong health. We want to change the way professionals practice so that they stop re-traumatizing people who seek care. We want to prevent children from being harmed and to reduce the impact when it occurs. We want to convince specialists to deal with whole people instead of just the parts presented for expert treatment. And we want to empower all of the Isaacs and those who love them to change society's priorities – to prioritize children's right to safety, to support their parents, and to demand compassionate health care.

Jon and I are pissed off. You should be too. Join us and let's start a Care Revolution.

JON AND I MEET in my office every Monday for an hour without an agenda. We are as likely to be talking about our families as comparing notes on challenging patients, planning a research study, critiquing the works of an obscure musician, or whining about a night on call. The conversation helps us both to do the work that often leads others to burnout – something we have been spared for the most part so far – and has allowed us to collaborate on the ideas that we have developed to try to help our patients and to teach our students, who are residents training to be psychiatrists, ideas that we have described in dozens of journal articles and several books.

Our Monday meeting is a reflective space, an invaluable opportunity to step back from the urgency of reacting to the demands of work that is busy, is full of uncertainty, and can provoke strong feelings. When we give ourselves space, and especially when we share our thoughts and feelings, things change. We are able to play with ideas, wonder about possible explanations for challenging problems, explore alternative perspectives, and enjoy a relationship in which we can each be fairly certain of acceptance, support, honesty, and respect from the other. Although the connotation is now obsolete, *revolution* once meant "consideration or reflection," like turning something over in your mind. So even our Monday meeting is revolutionary in a way. It's the best hour of my workweek.

Play, wonder, exploration, and *enjoyment* are rarely words that I would use to describe my time with Isaac. He sits in exactly the same chair as Jon does, in the same office, but the space between us is entirely different. It is rare to find moments when Isaac and I can play because play requires safety and security. That comes naturally for Jon and me, but for Isaac and me, it is an achievement.

I am going to tell a story of Isaac and me that is as authentic as I am able to re-create. And then we will talk about revolution; things need to change. But to get there, we need a reflective space in which to think about what it all means.

My time with Isaac often doesn't allow for much reflection. Reflecting comes afterward, on my own or in discussion with Jon. The book is organized to match that rhythm – conversations with Isaac, which are often intense and sometimes bewildering, alternate with reflections in which we explore the meaning and implications of his experiences and our work. Thus, the book's organization mirrors the structure of the type of thoughtful play that supports healing: facing Isaac's experience directly; allowing space for the emotions his memories bring; trying to make sense of it all by reflecting upon his experience and other experiences of which they remind us; creating stories, sometimes together, sometimes alone; and letting all of that thought, feeling, and *relationship* take our minds in unexpected directions.

In Isaac's email, he asked me to give everything that I have to help him deal with "the damage that I am." No half measures.

Here we go ...

2

"Fuckin' dead weight"

When Isaac first came to see me, I thought it was to get help coping with Crohn's disease. The psychiatrists at my hospital who treat people with physical illnesses had divided up the diseases between us, and Crohn's disease belonged to me.

Crohn's causes the gut to become swollen, painful, and dysfunctional, sometimes for long periods, often unpredictably. It means days with dozens of crampy, bloody, urgent bowel movements, nights lying awake with fever, sweat-soaked bedsheets, and pain. It comes and goes, often with no pattern. It is an invisible disease and elicits very little sympathy.

Isaac told me that parts of his intestine had been removed by a surgeon five times, each a few years apart. Usually, people with Crohn's disease take powerful anti-inflammatory drugs to control the disease. Some need surgery, but drugs are the mainstay. Isaac, on the other hand, wasn't taking any medication when he came to see me. He hadn't found it helpful. Instead, Isaac told me that he was prepared to manage his disease with repeated operations.

"I've done the math," he explained. "Each time they operate, they take out eight or ten inches of intestine. The operations have been five to seven years apart. My small intestine is twenty feet long. I'm forty-five. I have more intestine than I have years. Why take the drugs?"

The arithmetic was right, but I had never heard anyone speak of repeated major operations with such cold-blooded calculation. Isaac showed no hint of anxiety. He seemed to have a version of Crohn's disease that was resistant to the usual drugs, but it wasn't making him anxious, and as far as I could see, he wasn't depressed either. So why did he need a psychiatrist?

From the start, I saw Isaac's strength before he let me see anything else. And his strength was impressive. It wasn't just the surgery calculation, although that would have been enough to capture my attention. He was articulate, intelligent, a bit intimidating. He held a senior position in a large labor union. We spoke only briefly about his work, but he conveyed his passion for it, and I had the sense that he would be a tough opponent in a dispute.

His appearance reinforced the impression. He was skinny, but he didn't look weak. He wore a white dress shirt, a vest, a woolen tie, a pair of jeans that looked new, and well-worn cowboy boots. His gray hair was long and a bit unkempt. He had his own style.

Isaac looked around my office. At a first meeting, people often look around nervously, but he didn't look nervous. It was more like he was taking his measure of me and waiting for his moment. Then, very quickly, he caught me by surprise and told me why he was here.

"I'm living in an empty apartment with a cot and a shitty radio. I moved away from my wife three months ago. I haven't bought anything for the apartment. I don't know if I'm going back home."

"Why did you move out?"

Isaac hesitated and then spoke. He had been sexually abused as a boy and had kept it secret from everyone, including his wife, ever since. He had recently broken his silence, telling his wife, Sarah, what had happened. Her response had made him feel so hurt and angry that he left their home to find some space to regain his equilibrium. He regretted having told her, but now, having opened the subject, he needed to talk to someone.

I didn't know how to reply. Sarah had hurt him, and I didn't want to add to his obvious pain. I decided not to ask about the abuse. I asked, instead, what Sarah had said.

Isaac explained that she felt betrayed. Learning that your partner has kept a life-defining experience from you through twenty-five years of marriage would shock anyone, but at that point, Isaac wasn't up to thinking about Sarah's perspective.

Her response, "that explains a lot," made him feel small and then angry.

But the part Isaac could not forgive was that Sarah had told her girlfriend about it. I imagine she needed some support, but Isaac saw only a circle of expanding humiliation – gossip and sideways looks that would say "that explains a lot."

So, from the very first time we met, I saw Isaac's strength, and then I was invited into his most painful secret. He let me know that what made him feel safe was to be alone – by himself, with only a cot and a radio – but he also let me know that he could not survive without talking to someone. I was struck by the fact that he could be both a detached calculator of risks and a man so bound by shame. You could string a tightrope between those poles, so dramatic was the tension between them. In a sense, our conversations are about walking that tightrope, sometimes with grace, sometimes just clinging, trying not to fall.

I have never asked Isaac why he decided to trust me that day. But somehow, he decided that I would get a pass into the inner world that no one else was allowed to enter. It is a dark, confusing, painful, frightening place. Sometimes, however, trying to see the world through Isaac's eyes makes it seem more reasonable. It challenges the "difficulty" that I ascribe to him when he assaults a doctor, refuses a treatment that would relieve his suffering, or intimidates the dean of his son's university. The choices that make him seem dangerous and inexplicable to others make sense from Isaac's point of view.

NINE-YEAR-OLD ISAAC and his brothers, Neil, who is a year older, and Scotty, who has just turned six, are walking with their father past the rock garden, around the side of their house in a nice Bronx neighborhood. Isaac's father wears a suit, although it is a hot Saturday in July. He always wears a rumpled suit. I imagine it makes him look like an extra in *The Godfather*. He glances up, an unlit cigar gripped between his back teeth, and points down at the heavy ornamental ball and chain that decorates the wrought-iron gate.

"See that fuckin' ball and chain? That's what you are to me: fuckin' dead weight. Heh, heh, heh."

It's not the first time his sons have heard that comment; it's a favorite. That's one ACE: repeated, humiliating insults.

At fifteen, Isaac tells his dad he wants to go somewhere for summer vacation.

"You should hitchhike. Take Scotty with you. See the fuckin' world. Take a chance."

Scott is twelve. Isaac is short, skinny, and sickly, no match for whatever they might find on the road, and an unlikely protector for Scott. Their trip, hitchhiking across the Midwest, gets predictably complicated. That's a second ACE: lack of parental protection and support.

ACE number three is being hit by his father, sometimes for discipline, sometimes in anger. The fourth ACE: being raped by his next-door neighbor, repeatedly, over several years. A lifetime of living with the consequences of these harms is summed up by Isaac's ACE score – four.

Isaac scores a zero for the other categories. No one in his family had a mental illness or was too drunk or high to care for him and his brothers. They had clothes and food; money was not a concern. There was no violence between his parents, and they did not separate. No one went to prison.

Isaac's traumatic childhood has shaped his health. He has smoked since he was eleven. For most of his life, he has also used prescription and street drugs to change how he feels. As is typical of people with high ACE scores, Isaac is at high risk of serious diseases. An ACE score of four about doubles his risk of heart disease, increases his risk of chronic lung disease by a multiple of about four, and increases his risk of attempting suicide by a factor of six.

Isaac has nightmares and insomnia that trace a straight line back to his childhood and he has often insisted that one day he will die by suicide. He gets migraines and lives with pain in his joints and in his gut. His Crohn's disease, although not caused by trauma, emerged at the same age, so they are inextricably linked in his mind. It flares up in response to stress, which then causes more stress. Because of his childhood experiences, he is difficult for a medical professional to help. He doesn't trust easily, and he especially mistrusts doctors. Worse, many doctors have acted in ways that confirm that he is right to be wary.

MUCH OF DR. TRACIE AFIFI's career as a professor of psychology at the University of Manitoba has been dedicated to determining how often children are abused and how that relates to their adult health. In 2016, one of her studies, published in the *Journal of the American Medical Association* (JAMA) *Psychiatry*, got a lot of press, including on CBC. It reported that the rate of childhood abuse among members of the Canadian military was almost 50 per cent, compared to 31 per cent of the general population. Scrolling through the comments posted online, I noted a wide range of passionately held beliefs. One of the common responses is hostile skepticism:

> "Sounds like a B.S. study."
>
> "I was spanked as a child. I didn't kill or beat anyone during my military service. I haven't killed or beaten anyone since I got out 36 years ago."
>
> "I don't even believe the 31 per cent figure ... What is their definition of 'abuse'? The nice thing about statistics is that if you ask the questions the right way you can make them say whatever you want them to ... 'Figures lie and liars figure' and ... 'there are lies, damned lies and then there are statistics!'"

Someone else reflected on how what they once accepted as normal now looks like violence:

> "I got the belt from my father ... and was held against a wall and choked while my feet were off the floor ... My father was a lifelong service member, alcoholic and an abuse victim himself. His father was also in the military. I know that times were different then 'spare the rod ... etc.,' but when I look back at growing up on bases, I think that there was far more abuse ... and that we took it as normal. It wasn't until I was referred to a shrink that I realized just how violent our household was. Scary."

The commentator who asks for definitions has a point. Being spanked and being held against the wall by your throat are very different events. The commentator who came to see childhood experiences differently over time also has something to teach – we are not always reliable witnesses to our own experiences. A friend recently told me, "The only time I ever swore at my father, he knocked me off my feet. Not that it's okay to do that, but I learned not to cross that line." Her grudging respect for the lesson learned is common and is an attitude that leads people to be skeptical of the evidence that childhood harm by adults has serious long-term consequences. If you call it abuse, then someone is implicated. Maybe your father. Maybe you. It is hard for anyone to be objective.

So, we need to be clear about what we are talking about. Perhaps the most objective way to be clear is to ask, "What happened?" rather than, "Were you abused?" which requires a judgment about whether what happened counts as abuse. Then we can use the tools of science to see how what happened is linked to what happened afterward, including getting sick.

I use four ways to define and identify childhood adversity. The most objective method is to look at cases of abuse that are reported, investigated, and substantiated by law enforcement and child welfare agencies while the victim is still a child. I won't refer to these cases very often because they miss an enormous number of unreported events. Still, the impact of even this group is huge. An estimate of the economic burden of reported child maltreatment in the United States found the average lifetime cost was over $800,000 per person for kids who survived (it is much cheaper if the child dies). The total economic burden of investigated cases was $2 trillion. That is a lot of money for a drop in the bucket of child abuse cases. The authors of that study concluded that the cost was high enough that it "might offset the cost of evidence-based interventions that reduce child maltreatment." No shit.

Beyond the cases that are reported, we get a better sense of the magnitude of the problem by asking adults what happened when they were kids. Physical abuse and sexual abuse are the types of adversity that are most consistently linked with adult troubles. I will sometimes lump them together in one category: child abuse. Physical abuse is experienced by about one kid in four. Let that sink in: *a quarter of children are physically abused*. Using a representative study of these experiences, physical abuse includes being slapped on the face, head, or ears, or hit, or spanked with something hard three or more times (which occurs in 22 per cent of cases); being pushed, grabbed, or shoved, or having something thrown at you to hurt you three or more times (which occurs in 10 per cent of cases); or being kicked, bit, punched, choked, burned, or physically attacked at least once (which also occurs in 10 per cent of cases). A large portion of the one in four kids who are physically abused have experiences like the commentator who was getting the belt and being choked or like my friend who was knocked off her feet. Sexual abuse happens to about one kid in ten. It is defined as experiencing attempts or being forced into unwanted sexual activity by being threatened, held down, or hurt in some way, or experiencing unwanted sexual touching, grabbing, kissing, or fondling against your will. The third type of severe adversity is witnessing interpersonal violence at home. About one kid in twelve sees or hears their parents, stepparents, or guardians hitting each other or another adult in the home three or more times. The victim is usually a female parent.

Child abuse is gendered. Girls are more likely to experience sexual abuse and boys, physical abuse. Overall, just as Dr. Afifi reported, about one in three kids experiences at least one of these types of abuse by the time they turn sixteen. There is nothing subtle about this part of the story.

The third way to identify childhood adversity is broader. This is the concept of ACEs introduced by Vincent Felitti. In his original measure, there were ten categories of ACE events, which were added up to create each person's ACE score. The specific categories and their definitions are listed in the table below. ACEs and the ACE score are research tools that have demonstrated the link between the degree of adversity in childhood and myriad adult health problems over and over again. However, like many research tools for large-scale studies (Felitti's group surveyed more than twenty thousand adults), the ACE questionnaire sacrifices depth and breadth for brevity. The ten categories of ACEs are convenient for research, but they are not comprehensive. Although not in the original ACE questionnaire, growing up in a neighborhood that is unsafe is an ACE. Being bullied is an ACE. Being badly treated because of the color of your skin or your sexual identity is an ACE. Living in foster care is an ACE. Having a parent die when you are young is an ACE. And so on.

Of course, knowing that a kind of ACE, say, physical abuse, occurred is not enough. One needs to know *what happened* to appreciate its impact. One of the problems with ACE scores is that too many people have focused on the score rather than the kinds of experience that the score was trying to capture. Still, ACE scores are useful for raising awareness because ACEs are so common. Almost 60 per cent of people have experienced at least one of the original ten. Having experienced four or more, like Isaac, is a degree of exposure that markedly increases disease risk and occurs for about 15 per cent of people. A risk factor for illness that occurs in *so many people can have an enormous influence on the health of a nation.*

The fourth and final type of adversity that I refer to is more subtle. Some people experience the *consequences* of trauma without ever experiencing the trauma of physical or sexual abuse or having a high ACE score.

Types of Adverse Childhood Experience

	Before the age of eighteen
Physical abuse	An adult in your home often pushed, grabbed, shoved, slapped or threw something at you, or ever hit you so hard that you had marks or were injured.
Sexual abuse	A person at least five years older touched or fondled you, or had you touch their body in a sexual way, or attempted or actually had oral, anal, or vaginal intercourse with you.
Emotional abuse	An adult in your home often swore at or insulted you, or put you down, or acted in a way that made you afraid that you would be physically hurt.
Emotional neglect	Often feeling that no one in your family loved you or thought you were important or special, or that your family didn't look out for each other, feel close to each other, or support each other.
Material deprivation	Often not having enough to eat, or having to wear dirty clothes, or having no one to protect you, or your parents being too drunk or high to take care of you or take you to the doctor if you needed it.
Parental Separation	Parents separating permanently or divorcing.
Family member with mental illness	Living with someone who was depressed or mentally ill or attempted suicide.
Family member with substance abuse	Living with someone who was a problem drinker or alcoholic or who used street drugs.
Family violence	Witnessing violence against your mother or stepmother who was often pushed, grabbed, slapped, or had something thrown at her, or sometimes kicked, bitten, hit with a fist, or hit with something hard, or ever repeatedly hit for a few minutes or threatened with a knife or gun.
Family member jailed	Having a family member go to jail.

Additional evidence-supported types of childhood adversity

Being treated badly or unfairly because of your race or ethnicity; not feeling safe in your neighborhood; being bullied often; living in foster care; experiencing the death of a parent; having low socioeconomic status; having someone close experience a bad accident or illness; having parents who frequently argued; having no good friends.

So, some people are prone to stress-related illnesses, use coping strategies that increase their risk of disease, experience physical symptoms that are hard to explain and treat, and so forth, without having experienced obvious adversity. One reason for this is what child development experts call an *invalidating environment.* Some kids are raised by people who, for their

own reasons (often problems with depression or addiction, or the consequences of trauma in their own life), are not able to be as attentive and
responsive as is ideal.

Parents who are attuned to their kids' needs and respond fittingly
often enough (not always – the bar is not that high) help their kids to
develop in ways that keep them healthy – emotionally flexible, independent, sociable, reflective, resilient. Other adults who frequently and consistently interact with kids can also have an influence, but the ones who
do the parenting (whether or not they are biological parents) have by far
the greatest impact. Attuned and responsive parents are able to imagine
what might be going on in the minds of their little growing people and
respect their forming identity. That is what is meant by *validating*. The
absence of a validating environment leads growing children in a different
direction – either overly attentive to their parents (with "long antennae"
to detect their mental states and predict their behavior) or disengaged
(precociously independent, keeping everything inside). Neither strategy
is good for managing stress in the long run. The health effects of an
invalidating environment probably also depend on the kid's tempera-
ment. Some kids are born more sensitive; they thrive in an enriching and
validating interpersonal environment and may wilt in a stressful and less
responsive one.

These different kinds of adversity often go together. Physical and sexual abuse are almost certainly accompanied by a high ACE score and
very often by invalidating parenting. Not always though. Some people
who grow up fairly resiliently in spite of abuse or great losses may do so
because they have the good fortune to have supportive and responsive
parents to help them through it.

Isaac experienced physical abuse from his father, sexual abuse from
his neighbor, humiliating emotional abuse and neglect, and parenting that was inattentive to the point of providing a master class in
invalidation. I find it almost impossible to imagine how he could
have escaped the effects that each of these types of adversity has had
on his health.

3

Drowning

When I first met Isaac, my wife and I had our first two kids, boys. We would take turns dropping them off and picking them up as we traveled between work and home. The overpacked schedule of working parents tends to keep you focused on details: Who is doing pickup? Which kid is where?

Each day, I had to make a kind of mental commute as well as the physical one, because I do the kind of work that keeps your attention on the big picture. I listen to people talking about being really sick and dying and I try to be useful. My specialty, the psychiatry of the medically ill, is called *consultation-liaison psychiatry*, or often just CL. Like a lot of doctors who end up doing CL, I couldn't decide when I was training which I liked more, psychiatry or physical medicine, and then landed on the one that allowed me to pay attention to my patients' entire lives.

My specialty suits me. I have always been drawn to the idea that the most important challenges in life involve facing the realities of existence head on: accepting the inevitability of death, appreciating that the cost of freedom is responsibility for our actions, experiencing the unresolvable tension between living alone in your own skin and connection with others, and trying to create meaning in a universe that refuses to yield any. CL psychiatry is a practical application of that existential outlook. A colleague once said that CL psychiatrists are the "firefighters of despair," which may be too flattering but feels apt.

My office is cluttered with the stuff that makes it mine: books of phi-losophy and poetry, postcards from conferences where Jon and I have pre-sented our work, framed record albums, awards for this or that, two sets of stacking Russian dolls featuring images of the Beatles (each in the same order, John is on the biggest doll; Ringo comes last). The objects make it easy for patients to divert the conversation for a moment ("What's that?" "Oh, I like that album, too"), which helps sometimes with the kind of conversations we have. Two steps forward/one step back is a pattern that helps people keep their bearings.

Isaac was having none of that.

By September 2001, we had been meeting for over a year and our sessions had found a rhythm and a tempo that was dictated by Isaac's urgency to express himself. My job was mostly to listen, to say enough to let him know that I understood when I did, and to help him find words for the parts that were incomprehensible or unspeakable.

The week before the twin towers came down, Isaac was telling me about being assaulted when he was nine. We were working hard to find the right language.

It happened in his house. His mother had left him alone in the care of the young man who lived next door and who was ten years older than Isaac. Isaac was having a bath and the young man was with him. Isaac's mother was home, just not paying attention. That was not unusual for her. In later years, she said that she was not cut out to be a mother and didn't like it very much. Isaac couldn't be explicit about what happened in the tub. He remembered, but he couldn't say.

"It was completely irresponsible. She left me with him ... His face ... I could ..."

Isaac's expression contorted into a disturbing configuration. His feel-ings were intense, but the emotion could have been anything. Shame, rage, fear. I couldn't tell.

"I didn't know what the fuck was happening. He had me by ..."

"We have time. You don't have to talk about this if it doesn't feel safe. You don't have to go this fast."

"I've got to say this while I can ... I can't say it all yet. But I was going to drown. That's what I need to say. I was going to drown. I didn't know what was going on. I couldn't breathe."

Isaac never feels safe. A lifetime of insomnia and vigilance makes sense once you realize that nowhere is safe. A baseball bat under the bed makes sense too. Isaac sleeps better when his dog is beside his bed. He needs a dog or a baseball bat to sleep.

After 9/11, most people couldn't talk about anything but the attack. My patients focused on whatever angle matched up with their own vulnerabilities or preoccupations. Isaac flipped back and forth between memories and current events so fluidly that our conversation was a chaos in which every blurred detail seemed to matter.

"You've seen the footage of New Yorkers walking around Ground Zero looking dazed, not knowing what happened ... the ones all covered in the ash. I mean people who must have been blocks away, wandering around like zombies, not knowing where to go ... That's what it is like for me. I walk around saying, 'What happened to me? What is going on?'"

"Hmm."

"I could be a terrorist. No rules, just revenge. I could do that."

Isaac imagined unfettered aggression against oppressors. He objected when I phrased those thoughts as imagination, as a wish. He needed me to see that he was dangerous. The more time we spent together, the more I cared about Isaac. Part of him hated that. He didn't want to be someone to feel sorry for but someone to fear.

Growing up in an invalidating environment tends to leave a person insecure and mistrustful. To defend against hurt, Isaac had found that the best defense is a strong offense, which serves to keep others at a distance. Some respond to hurt and fear in the opposite way, seeking solace in close, dependent relationships, while fearing rejection and isolation. Both of these defenses are barriers to the kind of effective assertiveness that would encourage others to be supportive.

Fortunately, Isaac had figured out that it helps to talk about his dreams. That was a hopeful sign for me. Dreams are little creations. Unlike stark, traumatic memories, they give Isaac and me a place to play. Some people think their dreams are premonitions or that I am going to decode them like a secret message. That never really works for me, so I don't push patients for dreams, but if they find them curious and interesting, I'm in.

Isaac and I talk about his dreams like you might talk about a painting or a poem: something ambiguous that changes a little each time you see it.

He had a repeating dream in which he was drowning his mother in the backyard pool. Last time when he tried to drown her, she resisted. This time, she just let it happen.

I listened, trying to make sense of it. There was nothing subconscious about Isaac's rage at his mother. He blamed her for failing to protect him, for being indifferent to his well-being. But now, in his dream, he was drowning his mother much as the young man next door had done to him. So, he was identifying with his terrorist, hating the *victim* of the assault, the one who doesn't resist – himself.

Another day, another dream. There was a 30-foot python outside Isaac's room.

Isaac said, "I wanted a gun to shoot the dog."

The dog? I corrected him: "You meant snake, but you said dog. You said you wanted to shoot the dog."

"Huh?"

"Was there ever a dog, in real life, a dog that got shot?"

"Zero, our bulldog. He bit my brother Scott on the nose, so my granddad shot him. With granddad, you only got one chance."

Who was the protector, who the terrorist, who the victim in his dreams and memories? It was all getting blurred. It seemed that no one was safe. I felt like I was the one drowning.

Interactions that feel overwhelming to one participant in a conversation often feel similarly bad for the other. Sometimes that happens as we get closer to the important stuff. Writing about the Vietnam War, veteran Tim O'Brien made a similar point about the shame or embarrassment that people experience when he is blunt about what happened:

"You can tell a true war story if it embarrasses you. If you don't care for obscenity, you don't care for the truth ... Send guys to war, they come home talking dirty." Therapy with someone who has experienced childhood trauma feels a bit like that; it can make you feel dirty. I need to be able to live with my unease.

It wasn't just 9/11, traumatic memories, and nightmares that autumn. Isaac's Crohn's disease had been running out of control with pain and fevers for weeks. Twice Isaac had been in the Emergency Department with an obstructed bowel, an event that feels like having a horse kick you in the gut, having your stomach being pumped full of air like an overinflated tire, and being skewered up the ass, all at the same time.

Isaac's gastroenterologist had insisted that he start a new treatment, a drug that requires an intravenous infusion at a specialty clinic. During the second infusion, Isaac had an allergic reaction. His lips swelled, he became faint, and he found it very hard to breathe. The clinic staff treated the reaction, and the symptoms subsided, but in the meantime, Isaac felt like he was drowning again. The gastroenterologist was miles away, back in his own office, while Isaac was gasping for air. Although he didn't realize it, the experience was triggering memories.

Isaac raged into my office. "He was irresponsible, completely negligent. Unforgivable. He was completely indifferent. He orders these drugs but doesn't give a shit what they do."

But Isaac's disease needed to be controlled. He needed the doctor whom he could no longer trust. Intent on not alienating the specialist, Isaac worked hard to contain his anger for a couple of weeks and then he went to see him, a bit calmer.

Can you imagine if Isaac had seen the specialist at the peak of his rage? The gastroenterologist would feel wrongly accused and outmatched. I don't know many doctors able to defuse a conflict that formidable, especially when they have no idea where it is coming from. Even a doctor with strong communication skills could find it overwhelming. Empathy would fail; each would cut off the other, leaving each alone with his emotions. Exchanges like that are common for people with high ACE scores, whose experiences have taught them to be wary of harm or that the best defense is a preemptive first strike.

Being allowed into Isaac's world gives me a glimpse of what goes wrong in medical treatment and why. How could the specialist know how similar an allergic reaction could be to a sexual assault thirty years earlier: the sense of drowning, the absence of the person who "should have" protected him, Isaac's inability to control the threat himself? Without that knowledge, how could Isaac's gastroenterologist appreciate Isaac's rage? Even Isaac, in the midst of the events, doesn't connect the dots. Without that knowledge, the whole encounter between Isaac and the gastroenterologist just looks dangerous and inexplicable.

It is not hard for a specialist to ask about ACEs, but it rarely happens. Even a very simple conversation with few details shared is enough to convey that you are open to hearing more when and if it is relevant – that it is safe to talk. That short conversation can change the whole doctor-patient dynamic – it could be revolutionary – but instead there is usually silence.

I HAVE NEVER HEARD a colleague call a patient *hateful,* as in the title of the 1978 *New England Journal of Medicine* article, but patients like Isaac are often called *difficult.* It is a slightly softer word, but the meaning is essentially the same – and it isn't accurate.

One of the useful bits of that paper is that it locates the difficulty in the health care provider, not the patient. "Difficult patients" trigger a feeling that a health care provider doesn't like. If I am finding Isaac difficult, it is because our interaction has made me feel ashamed, afraid, enraged, helpless, or some other feeling that is hard to bear. My emotion extinguishes understanding and distances us. If I am feeling something so intense, chances are that Isaac is too, although not necessarily the same feeling. The permutations are almost infinite. Imagine Isaac is afraid and covers it up with anger that pushes me away so that he can feel safer. I feel angry back. But then I am ashamed to be angry at someone who doesn't deserve it and whom I am trying to help. He doesn't speak of the fear, nor I of the shame. In an interaction like that, each of us is too consumed with how we feel individually to appreciate the other's perspective, and we each locate the source of difficulty in the other. We lose empathy.

It is the interactions that are difficult, not the patients. If I find talking with Isaac difficult, it is my feelings, not his behavior, that tell me so. Health care providers who are finding their care of a patient thwarted by their own anger, for example, often implicitly ask, "What is wrong with this person?" But we should ask a different question: "What is going wrong between us?" As in any relationship conflict, the answers can be complicated.

Isaac's allergic reaction triggered a terrifying memory of drowning. He didn't recognize that he was remembering something. Instead, he attributed his feelings to the current circumstance, which was terrifying in itself. Those attributions carried with them some features that belong to the original event, in particular that the person in charge is absent, negligent, and uncaring. The gastroenterologist hadn't really done anything wrong. But if the two had met when Isaac's reaction was most intense, their interaction would be doomed. People who have experienced trauma are triggered by experiences that make sense when you know their past but can make no sense at all if you don't.

A useful starting point to understand a difficult and perplexing interaction with a patient is to assume that, at the bottom of it, the patient is afraid. That may sound simple, but it takes practice to remember in the heat of the moment. It is hard to imagine fear when what you are seeing is someone who rejects all your efforts to help or angrily blames you for their predicament. Nonetheless, it helps to imagine or, ideally, to find some reflective space to "play" with the idea that beneath all that, the patient is afraid of something.

Human beings react to fear by doing things to feel safer and more secure. In an interaction with someone who has the potential of either providing relief or doing harm, we have two fundamental tactical choices. The first choice is whether we approach or withdraw. We can draw closer to the other, figuratively or literally, by asking for help or support in one way or another, or we can distance ourselves, managing on our own and finding some space to calm down or sort things out. The second choice is whether to express or suppress our thoughts and feelings. We can share our distress, or keep it to ourselves.

These choices are connected to each other. For the most part, approaching another person to seek support when you are feeling distressed goes hand in hand with expressing some of your distress. That makes sense because expressing distress is a signal for others to help or at least to offer solace. Distancing yourself tends to go along with keeping those thoughts and feelings to yourself, maybe even appearing just fine, if you can pull that off.

People who feel secure make choices about who and when to approach and avoid quite flexibly. That secure feeling allows them to be nimble and selective about letting others into their inner worlds or keeping that to themselves while they get on with the business at hand. But fear can make any of us inflexible. We get stuck at one point along the approach/withdrawal and expression/suppression continuum. Usually, the choices we make about how to act with others when we are afraid are pretty strongly conditioned by experience. We return to what has worked best in the past and especially to what worked best when we were kids.

Very difficult health care interactions usually occur because patients who have experienced some kind of trauma get stuck, in their fear, in an impossible interpersonal position – both seeking and rejecting help, for example. In a romantic relationship, the same impossible tension can manifest in other ways – "I hate you. Don't leave me."

Isaac's interpersonal choices consistently favor distance. At the best of times, he is self-reliant, strong, and independent. He has been very selective about letting a chosen few into his inner circle. It is an adaptive response to a life that has taught him that the world is dangerous but that he is resourceful. In a situation that is more fraught, he doubles down. He moves into an apartment by himself. He maintains his distance with anger. He intimidates. He frightens ("I could be a terrorist. No rules, just revenge. I could do that."). He finds strength and safety in this anger.

It can be helpful to recognize these patterns. Imagining fear when all you see is hostility allows space for empathy, which can diffuse rage. I once watched Jon respond to a Code White (the public address announcement that is made in a hospital when a patient turns violent). A muscular, enraged man in a hospital gown was pacing the halls of a medical ward trying to pull out his intravenous line, cursing and flailing his good arm when anyone approached. He was surrounded by security guards who made sure the situation didn't get out of hand but who did not intervene directly.

"What's your name, buddy?" Jon asked.

"Jimmy."

"I'm Jon. What's going on, Jimmy?"

"I need to get the fuck out of here."

"Okay. Let me figure out what's going on so I can help."

"I need to get out."

"Getting out may be an option ... I just need to figure out what's going on. Do you know why you're here?"

"I got this." Jimmy shows Jon the infected patch of skin on his leg.

"Ouch! That looks bad. Is it hurting you right now?"

"No. It's better since I came in ... I just need to leave."

"I hear you, Jimmy, but I still don't know what's going on that you gotta go now. Can we sit down to talk about this so I can help you?"

"Okay, but not in that room. I can't go back in that room."

"Okay, let's sit over here."

Fifteen minutes later, Jimmy was calm. His doctor arrived and confirmed that it would be medically safe, though not ideal, for him to go back to the street. I walked away as the voice on the overhead speakers said, "Code White, 10th floor, all clear."

When we met later, Jon told me about their conversation. "He was shit scared. He woke up in a panic attack. He didn't know where he was. He was confused and thought his room was the morgue. He was either already dead, or somebody was going to make him dead. He was trying to get out of the hospital because he needed to get where he felt safer."

Jimmy lives on the street and no doubt has had many experiences that explain his fear. Jon's calm manner, his genuine wish to help, and his readiness to see that, more than anything, Jimmy needed to feel safe were what worked. Jon didn't make a diagnosis or give Jimmy a drug. It was his brief *relationship* with Jimmy that transformed the situation from one of conflict to one of problem-solving.

In the days after his allergic reaction, Isaac tried to understand exactly what was going on. He couldn't figure it out completely, but he could see that throwing a fit at his gastroenterologist wasn't going to help. He worked hard with me and on his own for two weeks to contain the intensity of his anger. My efforts to witness and then understand his rage, to respect the terror of feeling like he was drowning, could not diffuse the feelings quickly, as Jon's efforts did with Jimmy, but they helped, I think, enough that when he did meet with the specialist, he left the appointment feeling like they were back on track and that he could keep his inner world to himself, as he prefers.

4

"Cure sometimes. Relieve often. Comfort always."

Isaac missed an appointment. He sent an email later that day when he realized what had happened. He had been lying in his bedroom in the dark for over a day, after a migraine had left him too sensitive to light to go out. We rescheduled for the next day.

Isaac is often in pain. It comes in many forms. The pain of a bowel obstruction versus the pain of a three-day headache. Pain he can describe with an apt metaphor versus pain that renders him incoherent. Pain as a barrier to human connection versus pain as the currency of relationship, when talking about his pain brings us closer.

I arrived at the hospital before it was busy. There was almost no one in the lobby as I crossed to the coffee bar. The barista saw me coming. He had my usual large, black, dark roast ready by the time I got to the counter. I took the elevator to my department where the halls were empty, except for Isaac, waiting in a chair outside my office. He didn't look good. His clothes were uncharacteristically mismatched and rumpled. His gaze was aimed at the floor. I unlocked the door and gestured him inside.

"Go ahead and drink your coffee," he offered as he walked in.

I smiled, sat down in my desk chair, and set the coffee aside. The window behind me was letting in the red glow of the rising sun. Isaac squinted, though the light was far from bright. I got up and adjusted the blinds to make the room a little darker.

"I still have the headache. It's better, but I can't do anything yet. My head doesn't work. I feel so sick."

"You missed work, too, I guess."

At the union, Isaac spends a lot of his time making sure that people stick to their agreements, but he thinks of it in more adversarial terms: he fights for a living, standing up for people who need a protector. It is a good fit – he doesn't take crap from anyone, and he can keep his feelings to himself. He has been at it a long time and has risen in the ranks. On a practical level, the job usually allows him to work around his health problems.

"I couldn't go in, but it's fine," he said tersely.

I could see Isaac getting irritated. I think it was the note of sympathy in my voice that rubbed him the wrong way. I kept quiet.

He paused, and the irritation seemed to dissolve. His tone became matter-of-fact. "Someday it will be too much. I'll know. I can tell that I'm deteriorating. I'm not going to live like this forever."

I could see where this was going. We had talked about suicide before, and now we were talking about it again. It was as if Isaac needed to stake his claim that to live or die is his choice, that it is up to him.

Even as I write this, Isaac still considers suicide at times. Not yet, because he has obligations to his children. Also, not yet, because his quality of life has not crossed the line that only he can locate, but someday. At best, it recedes to a wish for the relief that dying through some other means will bring. Isaac reserves the right to die, not in the abstract but in reality, soon but not yet.

Talking about suicide raised a conflict for me. My first job was to listen well, to try to appreciate what he was saying and how difficult it may be to say it. My effort and my craft are all directed toward empathy. But when the subject is suicide, other imperatives intrude. I must keep my patients safe, if I can. I have legal obligations and professional standards to consider.

In psychotherapy, the quality of the relationship between the therapist and client is the single most powerful determinant of good outcomes. With Isaac, I must work to show empathy, to help him to understand his emotions and the impact of his actions on others. At the same time, I must maintain enough breathing space to offer more than just companionship.

I made a quick, silent assessment that Isaac's suicide risk was not imminent. The effort was enough to remind me that I have a stake in the outcome; if push comes to shove, I will come down on the side of keeping Isaac alive. Since these professional reflexes favor a different outcome than the permission Isaac wants, they screw up my empathy. For a moment, to stay with him, I had to fight the reflexes that told me to keep Isaac safe. My thoughts were very deliberate; I was almost saying to myself, *just listen*.

I don't know what I said next. It would have been contrived, revealing the effort of trying too hard to get it right.

"You're here for your kids. The pain isn't bad enough to end it yet. But in the end, it's your call." Something like that.

Isaac and I talked about his plan to take his life and his insistence that he had the right to choose. It was pretty much all we talked about for the rest of the session. And then, as Isaac looked over at the clock, acknowledging that we were wrapping up, he said, "It's weird. My headache is better right now. That has happened here before. I don't know why talking helps for a while sometimes."

There is a biological reality to what Isaac was experiencing. Just as being treated badly, being rejected, for example, is processed in the brain almost the same way that we process physical pain, so too can a good relationship literally be soothing. What happens between people affects our physical well-being. It isn't magic, and it isn't as strong as codeine, but relationships matter.

On that day, a bit of relief was good enough. Isaac had made the effort to see me and had shared thoughts that he knew could strain our relationship. He couldn't be sure that I would be able to hear what he needed to say. I couldn't be sure either. We could judge, by the lifting of his headache, that for a little while, we got it right.

THAT APPOINTMENT WITH ISAAC did not require any specific psychological interventions and no medication was prescribed. In important ways, it was not even psychotherapy that helped; it was "good old-fashioned medicine." To understand that, one needs to appreciate that medicine is not what it seems. Some of its most attractive versions emphasize its least common virtues. Unlike every episode of *House*, it is rarely about getting an uncommon diagnosis right. Contrary to almost every billboard and newspaper insert produced by hospital charitable foundations, it isn't usually about finding a cure. Its professionals are not usually heroic.

Of course, some diseases are cured, and the more the better. Many infectious diseases and an increasing number of cancers can be cured with treatments that are the result of scientific specialization, technology, and biological research. But, as health care professionals, we don't actually spend much of your money or our time curing diseases. They are spent on two much more common health problems: chronic diseases that chip away at a person's vitality over the years, and illnesses that elude any effective identification or treatment.

The distinction between disease and illness is important. Disease is a biological thing. It refers to molecules, cells, and organs that are not doing what they should – as in Crohn's disease. When Isaac's gut is inflamed because the disease is active, you can see it in the reddened inflamed inner bowel wall with an endoscope, in the thickening of the gut wall visible in an MRI scan, in a blood test, or with your own eyes in an operating room. Illness, on the other hand, is an experience. Illness is what it feels like to be sick. Isaac's experience of being tired and overwhelmed by pain is illness. When that experience is the result of uncontrolled inflammation in his gut, his disease is causing illness. A day in a dark room incapacitated by a headache and nausea is also an illness experience, but one that has few signs of its biological cause. Illness is often caused by disease. But almost as often, illness occurs with no discernable disease.

If you want to understand the core of health care, think less about cure and more about health management and suffering. Health care is so expensive because of the cost of treating *incurable* chronic diseases, like heart and lung diseases, arthritis, and dementia. One of the great medical successes of our lifetime, effective treatment for HIV, turned a predictably fatal disease into a chronic, typically non-fatal one. In health care, the more we succeed, the more disease our patients live with. What *could* reduce the burden of disease that we live with, and the cost of health care, would be to prevent chronic diseases and reduce the burden of *illness* that they cause. One of the keys to accomplishing those goals is hiding in plain sight; it is improving the *relationships* in which health care occurs.

AS OUR POPULATION AGES, most older people have more than one chronic disease, which makes the treatment of each one more complex. The treatment guidelines that specialists follow to provide evidence-based care typically assume that only one disease is present. There is rarely a road map for treating multiple diseases that work against one another. The complexity makes it harder to treat each disease effectively, so their impact on quality of life and costs is more than the sum of their parts.

From the patient's perspective, it is illness rather than disease that matters most. When seniors with multiple diseases were interviewed about managing their health, they spoke about feeling overwhelmed and drained, stretched, and tired of the pain, and that they had no control over their health. They expressed frustration at the difficulty of keeping medications organized and at the emphasis of doctors and hospitals on drugs. They complained that medical providers were each only interested in one piece of their health, not in them as whole persons. While most of these patients' health care providers thought their care was patient centered and collaborative, patients felt that it was the providers who called the shots and described instances of not being heard. Although I characterize my appointment with Isaac, in which I just did my best to listen well, and he felt a little better for a while, as "good old-fashioned medicine," these seniors' experiences would suggest that medicine has drifted quite far from that ideal.

But what about when illness occurs out of proportion to disease? It is very common; about one-third of the physical symptoms that a family doctor investigates are never explained by disease. In a specialist's office, a similar proportion of patients have the symptoms of that medical specialty without having any observable disease to explain them. Every specialty has its version of these so-called functional syndromes. A rheumatologist who treats diseases like rheumatoid arthritis and lupus also sees patients with chronic fatigue syndrome and fibromyalgia, whose pain, fatigue, and insomnia the specialist cannot explain biologically. A gastroenterologist is equally puzzled by irritable bowel syndrome; a neurologist, by non-epileptic seizures; everyone, by chronic pain. These symptoms and syndromes get no respect. They are said to be *psychosomatic*, or "all in the head," in spite of the lived experience of millions of people who would testify that they are real, with their location very much in the body.

Dr. Lawrence Kirmayer, a psychiatrist at McGill University, calls these unexplained symptoms "a social and clinical predicament, not a specific disorder," in that they represent "a situation in which the meaning of distress is contested." In this predicament, patients often seek the validation that comes with the diagnosis of a biological disease, whereas health care providers prefer psychological explanations, which unintentionally (and sometimes intentionally) are dismissive of a patient's experience. People who once experienced abuse or neglect, and are now trying to navigate the medical system to find relief from the symptoms with no clear explanation, face a double whammy. First, they have to deal with health care providers who are ineffective at providing relief or even explanation. What's worse, the invalidation of their perspective that is inherent in such interactions repeats an old insult. At best they are not helped; at worst, reinjured.

Rather than diagnosis, treatment, and cure, doctors and other health care professionals spend most of their time reassuring some patients that they do not have a disease, helping others to manage suffering that is not very well understood, or supporting them in disability that they cannot cure and trying to convince them to act in their own best interest (often unsuccessfully). This means spending a lot of time with patients who are much more concerned with illness than with disease. Health care professionals, who have been educated and trained in a system that privileges specialization, biology, and cure over holistic integration and care, often view this work as something that gets in the way of practicing medicine, rather than being its core.

It was not always this way. We would be well served to attend to five-hundred-year-old folk advice: "Cure sometimes. Relieve often. Comfort always."

5

"You're in it with me now"

In the first few months of therapy, I worked hard to keep up with Isaac's pace, even as I cautioned him to take his time. He described multiple events of sexual assault by the young man next door. He also told me about the onset of Crohn's disease. The belly pain, diarrhea, and fatigue that are typical of that disease started shortly after the assaults when Isaac was ten. He had no way of knowing that it was a second problem. It all blurred into one.

Although Isaac had felt trapped, terrified, and wordless at the time of the abuse, the feelings he was sharing with me now were different. He had a desire for revenge that he could barely contain. He felt angry and hopeless, as if by sharing his secret he had surrendered somehow. He felt humiliated and, when he talked about his disclosure to his wife, Sarah, betrayed. Although we focused on the abuse and the chaotic mix of emotions that went with it, he left no doubt that he loved his children, wanted to heal his marriage, and valued our growing relationship. The first time I saw Isaac cry, he was telling me that he just needed Sarah to love him.

They started marital therapy, but when Sarah revealed some mixed feelings about reuniting, Isaac went full tilt in the opposite direction. He furnished his apartment, took a road trip for a month, and then another trip into the country after he returned. I imagine that Sarah might have just seen defiance and rejection at that point. But what Isaac felt was despair. "I'm fucked up beyond repair. I'm so damaged."

Isaac agreed to try an antidepressant drug. He started reading books about post-traumatic stress disorder and about therapy. He was walking that tightrope between despair and hope or between seeking connection and running away.

Then he described his dreams.

> *I am a blind man being led down the street by my beloved dog. I am not afraid.*
>
> *I have a body in a bag in the back of my car. I dig a deep hole and bury it. I want to look at who is in the bag but decide against it.*
>
> *I am tied to a chair. Another man is tied to a chair beside me. We are tormented by a third man who is wearing a ridiculous costume.*
>
> *I am in a dark room surrounded by shapes that swarm like swallows or bats. They look like bats but they have big genitals. They swoop by my head, barely missing me. Then, the swarm swoops up and plasters itself at full speed against the wall. The splatter of the creatures smashed against the wall makes a silhouette – it is your face.*

The hair on the back of my neck stood up as Isaac described the final image of the fourth dream.

Dreams are always ambiguous, always open to multiple interpretations, partial explanations, and revisions. I try to treat them with the same respect and curiosity that any product of creation deserves. We quickly discovered that Isaac shared that attitude to his dreams. He liked it when we talked about them.

I offered Isaac this interpretation: "I wonder if those dreams are partly about what it feels like to come to therapy. Maybe I am just looking for positive signs, but a blind man who is led by a trusty dog could be an optimistic metaphor for that choice ... The body bag seems like some kind of darker mystery. Maybe you're not sure if you want to go there yet ... The guys tied up ... I don't know."

I was silent about the last dream. Although it is common for people in psychotherapy to dream about their therapist, it was unnerving to have my identity formed from smashed creatures that seem mostly to represent sexual abuse. Although I didn't say it, I was aware that I wanted to put a positive spin on that dream too – to align myself with the smashing of the creatures instead of with the bats themselves.

Isaac had another interpretation.

"The guy tied to the second chair is you. The bat things are you. You're in it with me now. You're another captive."

I came to understand that he was right. His interpretation combined the two opposing forces characterizing much of our relationship and the growing trouble I was feeling about it. On the one side is how the relationship benefits Isaac – he needs a confidante and a protector or just not to be alone. On the other side is Isaac's fearful expectation that anyone whom he brings into his world will become damaged. I already sensed that his fear held some truth; I didn't feel like I knew what I was doing. Things were moving so fast. I wasn't afraid of Isaac, but I didn't feel safe.

Isaac took another trip. He was away on business for two weeks. When he returned, he told me that, after using large quantities of Percocet for years (which was news to me), he had quit. He had gone out of town to get through the worst of the withdrawal by himself. And then he moved back with Sarah. He was ready to start again.

This is how I figure out if we are on the right track in therapy, always in retrospect. If a conversation relieves a headache, it was probably the right conversation. If Isaac chooses a relationship over drug dependence, we must have been doing something right. But none of that was planned. It was all I could do to keep up.

JON AND I WERE in the same class in medical school in the 1980s. We were both on the Meds rugby team – I as a not very adept back, he as the coach because he had already blown out his knee. We had different friends, so we didn't sit near each other in lectures. I didn't get to know him very well until we both graduated and started training in psychiatry.

Now, we can reflect on our shared experience of being surprised to discover how much of the work of a psychiatrist involves attending to the traumas experienced by our patients. Neither of us made this discovery while in medical school, or even while we were training in psychiatry, but rather after a few years of practicing the specialty. Hence the surprise. Our education did not forewarn us; no one told us what we were getting into.

We had one lecture on "battered child syndrome," which introduced us to a 1962 paper by Dr. Henry Kempe and his colleagues. Kempe's was the first medical paper that described how to recognize the telltale signs of children who had been beaten when they presented to the Emergency Department (old, healed broken bones on X-rays, head injuries, and so forth). It was a groundbreaking report, although, in retrospect, the prevalence of such cases that they discovered was laughably low – 302 cases appearing in seventy-one hospitals in one year. Dr. Kempe would have been shocked to learn that one in three kids experiences serious physical and sexual abuse.

We probably had a lecture on the social determinants of health. It would have been mixed in with a bunch of community medicine lectures that shared space in the schedule with nutrition. The idea that early childhood experiences are strong risk factors for disease and illness was fully absent. Of course, we didn't notice anything was missing – as two guys with ACE scores of zero, we had neither experience nor book learning to draw our attention to the issue. Even in psychiatry, where in retrospect it seems to take an active process of avoidance not to notice how early trauma is connected to the bread and butter of our daily work, it was not a prominent idea (outside of the psychoanalysts who like to talk about the influence of childhood but seemed fixated on breastfeeding and fanciful theories of body parts becoming diseased to symbolically express forbidden thoughts ... it's amazing that we have ever been of any use to anybody).

So, we knew nothing about adversity and health. But we knew a thing or two about the difference between doctors and patients. We learned it from what is now called the hidden curriculum. In the eighties in medical school, just about everyone read *The House of God*, a novel about life as an intern by Dr. Samuel Shem. Its satire relieved the overwhelming anxiety that we felt about caring for patients at a time when we were sure that we were incompetent imposters. Much of its comedy relied on drawing a thick line between the book's protagonists – young doctors like we wanted to be, mostly male – and their common problem, patients. The dehumanization of the patient was suggested by slang terms like "gomer" ("a chronic problem patient who does not respond to treatment" according to the Merriam-Webster dictionary), which stands for "get out of my emergency room." The dehumanization was further reinforced by the doctor's solution to the problem, which was to turf the patient to another service. This was expressed by setting the patient's bed a little too high ("orthopedic height," from which a fall could break a hip) or a lot too high ("neurosurgical height," from which the damage would be greater), the result being that the patient becomes someone else's problem. It feels a little shameful to acknowledge that we laughed, but we did, and those words are still in the medical lexicon.

Of course, like all satire, the problem is not *The House of God* but the world it was satirizing. There is a very long tradition of health care professionals, especially but not exclusively doctors, maintaining distance to protect against being overwhelmed by human tragedies. This gets carried to an extreme when we professionals start to think and act as if we are actually different from our patients – as if the difference between us and them is anything more than expert training, and because we, unlike our patients, may not be sick, at least not at the moment.

Today, trainees are encouraged to write notes in which what they see is called *objective* and what their patients tell them is called *subjective*. They are taught to use unnecessary jargon, for example substituting *has suicidal ideation* (or worse, just *SI*) for "is thinking of killing himself." The jargon separates them from those who speak plain English, and it distances them from their patients' experiences. We routinely read notes written by young doctors in which they report (as they have been taught to do) that a patient "claimed" X and "denied" Y, rather than just writing that X happened and Y didn't. Their default position is to not risk fully believing what they have heard.

All of this is utter bullshit. A doctor's observations are just as subjective as a patient's, but from a different perspective. We have no way of knowing when our patients are telling the truth, and when they are not, but they are almost always trying to. We will all be fooled from time to time, but the value of starting by believing is far higher than its costs.

Beyond being nonsensical, distancing ourselves by distinguishing between us and them is dangerous for both patients and doctors. For patients, this distance, or in its extreme forms, objectification or dehumanization, devalues their actual experience or renders it irrelevant. When their childhood experience is the cause of their illness, distancing sets up a conversation in which the key to the puzzle is invisible or off limits. For doctors, fractured and impersonal relationships with patients contribute to ineffective practice and to burnout. It harms everyone.

MEMORY HAS A WAY of turning multiple events into one. So, the things I think I learned about Jon's father at his memorial service were probably acquired over a longer time. In my mind, however, the service marks our transition from acquaintances to friends. Jon's dad was R.C.A. Hunter, the esteemed chair of the Department of Psychiatry at the University of Toronto from 1967 to 1974. When he died in 1987, there was a large memorial at the university. I walked to the campus from Mount Sinai Hospital, where Jon and I were both in our second year of residency. I listened to my mentors speak with admiration about one of theirs. I learned that R.C.A. was a bombardier in the Royal Canadian Air Force in World War II, shot down over occupied Europe and imprisoned in a German prisoner of war camp, and that he didn't speak of what happened there. I learned that he influenced the department in which I was being trained toward a greater recognition of the interaction between biology and experience that causes mental illness. And I watched Jon cry as he tried to get through reciting his father's favorite poem, Yeats's "He Wishes for the Cloths of Heaven."

Had I the heaven's embroidered cloths,
Enwrought with golden and silver light,
The blue and the dim and the dark cloths
Of night and light and the half-light;
I would spread the cloths under your feet:
But I, being poor, have only my dreams;
I have spread my dreams under your feet;
Tread softly because you tread on my dreams.

Jon and I talk about these things now in a way that we did not at the time of his father's death: his father's war experience, R.C.A.'s influence on Jon, his parents' romance, which I recently learned about at his mother's funeral, Jon's losses, my dad's disappearance into Alzheimer's disease, the burden of his decline on my mother, the families of our parents and our wives' parents, all with their own ACEs, how these things creep into dreams and sometimes nightmares ... Everyone has these stories. There is no distinction between us and them.

And yet, even though I insist that there is no distinction between us and them, when Isaac tells me, "You're in it with me now," my reflex is to pull back from that idea and find comfort in so-called objectivity, to think about his dreams, not to participate in them. Like all reflexes, it is a protective move.

When we talk about it later, Jon tells me that, in fact, Isaac nailed it. "You're in. He wants you in, probably needs you in, but he's afraid for you. You earned your way in, and he's better off for you being there, but he's horrified by the prospect that you can be harmed like he was. You've done a difficult therapeutic thing here, and it is working and good for Isaac, but he knows what an awful place he's put you in. Hang on, buddy."

I sit back and let my shoulders drop. Having Jon in my corner allows me to do better work with Isaac. Every doctor should be so lucky.

6

"The closest thing to love"

Isaac often looks like he has something on his mind from the moment he walks into my office. Sometimes, after I sit down, I say, "How are you?" to start the conversation. Sometimes I just wait. Either way, he lets me know what he needs to talk about. This time he took a little longer to collect his thoughts.

"I had to talk to Simon. It was the hardest conversation I've ever had with him. He's not just my doctor, he's a friend." Simon was his family doctor and a friend of mine as well. "Did I ever tell you that we knew each other in New York? He's from my neighborhood."

"What did you need to talk to him about?"

"I faked a prescription for fifty Fiorinal. The pharmacist saw that I had forged his name. They called his office. I had to see him right away to talk about it."

Fiorinal is a painkiller, although not a common one. It is an old-school treatment for migraines, a combination of aspirin, caffeine, and a barbiturate. Aspirin is bad for Crohn's disease. Barbiturates are addictive; they are sedatives and muscle relaxers. They don't have much use these days.

We talked about the forged prescription for a while. It was unexpected and it was serious. The guy who found it so hard to trust others was making himself hard to trust. Had he done it before? No. Was he hoping to get caught? He didn't think so, he just needed the drug. What did Simon say?

"He didn't tell me to find a new doctor, which is what I expected. He took it seriously. He talked about an addiction clinic but I don't want that. He said he was going to monitor my prescriptions more closely. No painkillers or small prescriptions if absolutely necessary. I was relieved that he'll still see me."

I could feel my furrowed brow start to relax a bit after hearing that Simon had a plan. "Why Fiorinal?"

"Didn't I ever tell you that story?" Isaac settled in. "I was thirteen. I was having another migraine. They were relentless. I took the day off school. I didn't even ask my mother, I just told her. I never asked. She didn't give a shit."

Isaac grinned.

"She acted all worried at how sick I looked and said, 'Let me help you. Here, take my medicine.' She gave me the Fiorinal she took for her headaches. It felt great, the best feeling I ever had. She always had this giant bottle of Fiorinal. After that, she gave them to me whenever I said I had a headache. And I just helped myself whenever I wanted that feeling. That was when I realized how great drugs can be. It was the best fucking thing she ever did for me. I'm serious."

In individual psychotherapy, you get half of every story at the most. I try to remain aware that the others who I hear about are not just villains or victims. They have their own stories. Try as I might, though, it was hard not to conclude that giving a thirteen-year-old with a bad headache an addictive sedative was an act of exceptional negligence. The expression on my face probably gave away my reaction.

"Was she, uh ... was she just trying to make you better?"

"It was expedient. She just wanted the problem to go away."

"It was a different time. I don't know if they appreciated the risks in ... what was it, '67 or '68?"

"She didn't care. Look, the point is that it was great. It changed my life. It was the first time I had something that made me feel better."

Fiorinal became Isaac's favorite drug. Over the years, he has used a lot of drugs to change the way he feels; sometimes any change is an improvement. He has come off of drugs at times too, like when he moved back in with Sarah. When he stops taking drugs it is because he thinks that is best. When he takes them, it is usually because he wants an anesthetic. What doesn't change, whether Isaac is using drugs or not, is his love for them. And nothing could touch Fiorinal.

"It was the closest thing to love she ever gave me."

KIDS KNOW FROM EXPERIENCE about relationships and pain. The good version of that happens when the sting of a scraped knee is relieved when a parent or grandparent kisses it better. Isaac is also attuned to how personal relationships and pain influence each other. He notices when a conversation with me temporarily relieves a headache, and he appreciates his mother using Fiorinal as the debased currency of love.

Neurobiological research is catching up. An experiment has demonstrated the shared biology between rejection and pain. Imagine playing a game of virtual catch: just you and two ghostly, featureless cartoon figures on a computer screen throwing a digital ball back and forth, back and forth. And then something happens; the two cartoon figures start passing the ball between themselves, leaving you out. In the original experiment, you would have been told that the cartoon figures are operated by two real people in a different room. When they stop playing catch with you, the exclusion is personal. Later, the researchers determined that it doesn't matter, even being rejected by featureless cartoon figures that you know are not real still feels like something. It is the mildest version of rejection that I can imagine. The game isn't much fun in the first place and the cartoons are obviously not people, but those who participate in the experiment report that this small sting hurts.

What makes this minor social injury interesting is that the experiment is done while you are in a functional magnetic resonance imaging (fMRI) machine, which tracks what is going on in your brain as you play and as you recover from the sting of exclusion. The results of the imaging, first published by Naomi Eisenberger, a professor in UCLA's Department of

Psychology, and her colleagues in the prestigious journal *Science*, are intriguing. The fMRI images display a cross-section of your brain in which the parts that are actively working light up like bulbs on a Christmas tree. If you were to experience a physical pain like a pin prick or a burn while in the fMRI machine, the part of your brain that would light up is its "alarm detector" (the anterior cingulate cortex), the brain region whose specialty is detecting that something is wrong. That is exactly the part that lights up when you are excluded from the boring game of virtual catch. Shortly after a physical pain, the next brain part that would light up is the area whose job it is to turn the alarm off (the right ventral prefrontal cortex). The sequence that is observed after social rejection is exactly the same, first the anterior cingulate, then the right ventral prefrontal cortex – alarm and then inhibition.

Eisenberger's explanation is that social bonds are so important to adaptation and survival that, in the course of evolution, mammals have piggybacked the regulation of feelings related to social exclusion onto the neurological machinery that regulates physical pain. "Hurt feelings" are not just metaphorical.

The similarity between the biology of close relationships and of our interactions with the physical world is also found elsewhere in our brains. Thomas Insel, former director of the National Institute of Mental Health in the United States, has written about how the neurobiology of close personal relationships has piggybacked onto neurological circuits that are crucial to understanding addiction. The first of these neural circuits are those that are active when we experience pleasure. They represent the biology of liking some experiences. The biology of liking things is complicated, of course, but the part that is relevant to our story is simple: opiates feel good. The opiate chemicals we produce naturally, called endorphins, are released during pleasurable activities like having sex or eating chocolate. They are the chemical substrate of the long-distance runner's high, and they control pain. Opiates administered after surgery also reduce pain, or at least disconnect us from the distress it causes.

The second of the neural circuits are those that help us to find what we want. The biology of wanting, Insel writes, is mediated by brain circuits in which the nerves communicate with one another using the molecule dopamine. These so-called dopaminergic circuits detect what matters to us; they predict reward; they are beacons that point toward things we like and need. Substances that stimulate dopaminergic nerves, such as cocaine, are addictive. Insel suggests that it is these dopaminergic circuits that are responsible for crossing the line from liking how a drug feels to compulsively wanting it, which is the mark of addiction. Indeed, those with addictions often report that they have long lost any sense of enjoying the substance that they consume; they simply need it. The shift from liking to wanting or needing a romantic relationship is similar and is most starkly and painfully observed after rejection, when checking on an ex-partner or calling them becomes compulsive. The dopaminergic beacon wants what it wants, whether it is cocaine, a slot machine, or lost love.

Isaac's relationship with pain and pain medication has so many layers that it is hard to appreciate his experience as a whole. Let's peel back six of these layers. The first is physical pain, which has an obvious cause: Isaac's Crohn's disease. The same disease sometimes prevents his gut from working well, causing a painful obstruction. So, Isaac is often in severe pain from a mechanism that is not mysterious at all – a body part is harmed, and pain-detecting nerves in the tissue of that body part are triggered and relay their signal to the brain.

The second layer is physical pain that is real but from a source that is harder to identify. The many brain circuits that detect and manage pain are complicated. As Eisenberger's experiment shows, some can be triggered by personal events just as easily as they can be by pin pricks, burns, or bowel spasms. Other evidence shows that pain circuits in the brain can continue to reverberate and perpetuate the experience of pain (*illness*) long after an injury to the body's tissue (*disease*) has healed. Illnesses like irritable bowel syndrome and fibromyalgia can involve severe pain for which the source may be in the brain or spinal cord rather than in the parts that are identified as hurting. Beyond that, people who experience chronic pain often find that it is amplified by cognitive and emotional states including depression and anxiety. Indeed, antidepressant drugs sometimes reduce chronic pain, even for people who experience pain but are *not* depressed. These are layers within layers – the many ways in which real physical pain occurs for reasons other than the firing of a pain-detecting nerve in the gut or a muscle or a joint.

Isaac is often frustrated by doctors who find that the results of their tests do not fit with the degree of pain that he experiences. This introduces the third layer of complexity in his experience of pain, which is not being believed. People who have not experienced severe pain with an unclear cause often think that such pain is not real – that it is the result of faking, or seeking attention, or the inability to tolerate mild discomfort. Doctors, unfortunately, are not exceptions to this belief. Since pain is an internal experience, there is no objective measure to say which party in the dispute is correct. Having spent a career listening to people talk about pain, I am convinced by their reports. Of course, there are fakers in the world, but mostly people talk about pain because they feel it. Some exaggerate and some minimize, but few make stuff up.

Not being believed is toxic. For Isaac, disbelief almost always triggers rage and sometimes hopelessness. Disbelief is a kind of rejection. Eisenberger's experiment suggests that rejection by someone charged with providing relief could actually make the pain worse. Psychologically, it is invalidating. It is the second hit of the double whammy we described in Chapter 4, in which people whose physical pain is amplified and perpetuated by the psychological and neurological consequences of childhood adversity experience the reinjury of their perspective being undermined once again.

The fourth layer of complexity in Isaac's relationship with pain and anesthesia is that he *loves* Fiorinal. He *needs* it to treat his pain. The story would be simpler if he just needed it. But he is very clear that he also *likes* how it feels. He would take it if he were not in pain and sometimes does. "It changed my life. It was the first time I had something that made me feel better." He likes Percocet and codeine too, but he loves Fiorinal.

Layer five: Isaac relies on doctors to prescribe the drugs he needs for pain relief. They decide if a medication like Fiorinal or Percocet is advisable and how much is too much. The power imbalance between the two – the doctor's professional obligations, Isaac's dependence on his doctor – is rarely starker than in the moment that the doctor pulls out the prescription pad or refuses to. The stakes are high. Before the epidemic of deaths from powerful synthetic opioid street drugs, like fentanyl, which started in 2015 or 2016, by far the greatest number of opioid-related deaths were from prescribed drugs. Doctors are gatekeepers of both the benefits and the harms of these drugs, and the roles of gatekeeper and of care provider can conflict. Inadequate prescribing can be both safe and cruel. For Isaac, it has consequences that go beyond his experience of pain. He doesn't usually forge a prescription (this was the only instance as far as I know), but he has sometimes bought what he needs on the street. "Why should I risk being arrested to get what I need, just because a doctor has decided that I don't need it?" he has asked. It is a fair question.

The sixth layer is at the center of the onion. This is where we find the relationships in which Isaac will be believed or not, get a prescription or not, find a listening ear or not – the relationships in which he seeks understanding and solace. They are all based on trust. Simon counts on Isaac to do his best to describe what is really going on. Isaac counts on Simon to respond in good faith. Isaac has a lifetime of experience that teaches him to be cautious about trusting those who have authority over him. When he violates that trust, as he did with Simon, it threatens an alliance that has taken a long time to build and maintain.

Biology, interpersonal psychology, messy transactions in the real world, memories of harm and of terror, the oversight of professional bodies and of the law, and a fleeting chance to feel better ... Isaac's experience of pain and of the drugs he needs is almost hopelessly complex but also very common. I share those layers with him when we speak of pain and of drugs, which we do a lot. We agreed near the start that I will never prescribe pain medication to him and he will never ask. We've stuck to that pact. I couldn't manage the conversation if I was the gatekeeper to the drugs as well. I couldn't listen well enough if I was also evaluating, deciding, providing, or withholding the thing that feels like love.

7
Cause of causes

Isaac had his first cigarette when he was eleven.

The young man next door, a sexual predator, had grabbed him as he walked between their houses and dragged Isaac to the basement of the neighboring house in the Bronx. What happened next followed a pattern that had been established previously and would be followed many more times afterward. Isaac's clothes were off him almost as soon as he got downstairs. Being naked trapped him: helpless, ashamed, and resigned to what would follow. More happened. In the end, the young man ejaculated in Isaac's mouth and on his face. The effect of this was overwhelmingly frightening.

The effect was more malignant because of what the young man said next. Sometimes he said, "Someday you'll do this. This is what everyone does." Other times, "Your mother does this too." This particular time, he said, "What I did is nothing compared to what I will do to your mother if anyone ever finds out about this." Then he threw Isaac's clothes at him and told him to get out.

Isaac's house was lively when he entered through the side door. They had company, and no one paid any attention to his entrance. He had only one thought, *They're going to smell it. They're going to know.* He brushed his teeth for ten minutes and then put soap in his mouth, drinking and spitting out mouthful after mouthful of suds, careful to swallow nothing. All the time that he was frantically cleaning the he-did-not-know-what from his mouth, Isaac was thinking about what to do next.

Then he had an idea. He snuck down the hall from the bathroom into his mother's room and found a pack of smokes on the dresser. Kents. He stole what he needed, borrowed the lighter that sat beside the pack, went back into the bathroom, and smoked his first cigarette. He figured that his parents, both smokers, wouldn't detect the smell of cigarettes on him and wouldn't care if they did. His secret would be safe. Since then, Isaac has been a smoker.

I have usually just accepted that Isaac smokes, but today we are talking about it. Once again, he surprises me.

"You know, every time that I have lit a cigarette, I go through a checklist in my mind: 'Oh yeah, this is what it feels like. I love the feeling. I remember that feeling. I remember my first cigarette. It was a Kent. Why a Kent? Oh, yeah, I got it from the dresser. It was my mom's. Why did I steal a Kent? Oh, yeah, it was ... Oh, fuck. Oh, fuck.'"

Isaac looked horrified for a few seconds and then his expression relaxed. I shifted in my seat, absentmindedly holding the identity badges on the lanyard round my neck like a deck of cards between us.

He moved from the memory, which still has the power to discombobulate him, to contempt at his parents' indifference.

"They didn't have a clue."

"I'm stuck thinking about you in the bathroom in a panic. You really believed his threat."

"Of course I did. I figured he would kill my mother if I told her."

"You also figured out a solution, which was pretty impressive problemsolving under the circumstances."

"I had to do something."

"And I'm thinking about Fiorinal."

"Why?"

"You got them both from your mother. Your two substances. Cigarettes and Fiorinal."

"That's true. But she gave me the Fiorinal. I took the Kents. It was different."

"Yes. And I don't know if it matters or not, but you stole them both from her. You took what you needed from her. And you still smoke, even though it is bad for Crohn's."

"That's what they say, but I don't notice it. When I am up at night, I smoke. That is when it is best. I have a dream or I can't sleep. I just sit in the front room and smoke."

"Does it focus you or help you calm down?"

"I don't know, but I need it. And I don't care if it is bad for Crohn's. I'm not going to make it anyway. It doesn't matter."

He paused.

"Everything changed when I was in high school."

"Still in New York?"

"Yeah, yeah, same neighborhood ... I wasn't scared of anything. I took a lot of drugs. I was the toughest little shit in that school. I was feared and admired. I was four foot nothing and skinny and I always felt sick. But I had a girlfriend in the next grade up. She was out of my league, but she liked me. I skipped classes and smoked and took drugs that other kids hadn't heard of yet."

"You were learning not to look scared, I guess."

"I just wasn't scared. The drugs were really good." Isaac laughed.

I waited.

"You know I drove a cab when I was sixteen."

"What?"

"I had just got a driver's license I guess; I don't remember. But I knew how to drive before I had a license. And I went to this guy who had a few cabs and told him I could drive at night."

"And he let you?"

"He didn't give a shit. Or maybe he hesitated. But I could talk anyone into anything then. So, I drove. I learned every place in my part of the city. It was good."

"And dangerous."

"I had a tire iron that I tucked under the seat at my left hand. I was ready. You had to be ready."

"And you were small for sixteen."

"I sat on something that made me look taller. I wasn't scared. I was really tough. Can you imagine if it was your kid? But I had a tire iron beside the seat in case there was trouble. Sometimes there was."

I pictured one of my sons driving a cab in the Bronx at sixteen. "Jesus."

ACES ARE STRONG RISK FACTORS for disease. They increase the risk of many diseases, in some cases by a large amount. Generally, the risk of disease goes up in steps; the more ACEs a person reports, the more likely they are to have a serious disease. Comparing the risk of disease between people who had had none of the original ten ACEs (around 40 per cent of adults) and those having experienced four or more like Isaac (about 15 per cent), the risk of diabetes, heart attack, coronary artery disease, stroke, and asthma is about 50 to 100 per cent higher in the latter group. Childhood abuse in particular increases the likelihood of an adult having arthritis, back problems, high blood pressure, migraine headaches, chronic lung disease, and cancer.

The reason that the list of diseases that follow childhood adversity is so long and that some of the risks are so high is that childhood abuse and other ACEs don't cause diseases, they *cause the causes* of diseases. There is a cascade of risk in which the original insults to a child's safety and enrichment trigger a multitude of consequences, which trigger further consequences, which interact with each other, reinforcing and amplifying the processes that cause disease. The dominoes of disease causation fall like the actual dominoes in one of those complex demonstrations where one domino knocks down another, which triggers two or three lines of dominoes, and so on until there are dominoes falling in all directions.

The first contribution to that cascade is illustrated by Isaac's story. As children with high ACE scores grow up, they are more likely to do things that are risky for health. They are more likely to smoke and take drugs, to drink too much, and to get sexually transmitted infections. Of course, teenagers with high ACE scores usually don't have reasons that are as clearly related to adversity as Isaac's reason for smoking. It is more likely that they smoke or vape because it helps them to manage distressing emotions or because they fall in with a peer group that smokes. Isaac not only liked the feeling he got from drugs but also benefited from the image of being "the toughest little shit in school" who used a lot of drugs. Often, substances that lead to addiction start as a remedy to feelings of panic or depression or pain and become a problem only after they have been used as a remedy for a long time. For some, smoking or using other substances feels normal because their parents do it, or they don't have the kind of relationship with their parents that would help them oppose peer pressure. Beyond that, people with high ACE scores may be more drawn to drugs, including nicotine and alcohol, because their early experiences have altered the function of brain systems that control liking and wanting, as I described in Chapter 6.

The reasons are many and varied, but the relationship is strong. In one study, each type of adverse childhood experience on its own increased the likelihood of smoking. Those with an ACE score of five or more were almost three times as likely to smoke as those with an ACE score of zero. And then, of course, the dominoes fall. Smoking increases the risk of heart and lung disease, many cancers, and so on. Similar factors lead to earlier and greater alcohol use, which increases the risk of liver disease, motor vehicle accidents, high blood pressure, heart disease, stroke, some cancers, and a host of mental illnesses.

Growing up with physical or sexual abuse or in an emotionally invalidating family, or with other kinds of adversity, unsurprisingly, also shapes subsequent sexual experiences in a variety of ways. Isaac has very specific fears about being touched in certain ways that trigger traumatic memories – his intense startle reaction has caught Sarah by surprise and often leads him into an inarticulate shame-filled retreat in which he just looks angry and unapproachable.

For someone else, the consequences may be very different: seeking sex instead of love or in search of love, recurrently being in situations where the risk of sexual violence and exploitation is high, not feeling worthy of respectful treatment, valuing connection more than safety ... the possibilities are many. From a health perspective, many of these experiences increase the risk of unplanned pregnancy and of sexually transmitted infections. A survey of thousands of adults in Washington State found that those who experienced childhood sexual abuse were more than five times as likely to report that in the previous year they had used intravenous drugs, been treated for an sexually transmitted infection, tested positive for HIV, or had unprotected anal sex. Taken together, the risk of intravenous drug use and of sexually transmitted infections markedly increase the risk of potentially life-threatening infections like HIV/AIDS and hepatitis C.

People with high ACE scores die younger than those who grow up with less adversity, sometimes a lot younger. One study found that those with ACE scores of six or more died twenty years younger, on average. Another study, finding a strong, graded relationship between ACE scores and early mortality, concluded that exposure to childhood adversity leads to "radically different life-course trajectories." Perhaps surprisingly, the health burden of smoking more, drinking more, and other risky behaviors doesn't account for all of this early mortality. Nor is it accounted for by social determinants of health, which may accompany high ACE scores – poverty or parents' limited education or other indicators of social class. Evidence suggests that beyond these contributors to disease and early death, childhood adversity has direct biological effects. Very stressful experiences early in life can alter our biology, particularly when these events occur in key developmental periods, when the biological systems that regulate how we adapt to our environment are taking shape. Many chronic diseases are the result of poor regulation of intricate systems of physiological checks and balances that control immunity and other aspects of adaptation to our environment. ACEs alter the development of these systems, leaving them not so finely tuned and prone to diseases of wear and tear, like many cardiovascular diseases.

Even at the level of individual cells, extremely stressful early experiences impair health. This can be measured by the length of telomeres,

which are the end parts of chromosomes, the protective caps that prevent various types of damage to genes. At the start of a cell's life, the
telomeres on its chromosomes may comprise eight thousand to ten
thousand pairs of the nucleotides (the genetic alphabet) that form the
backbone of DNA. Every time the cell divides, the telomere is shortened
by a bit until it becomes too short to do its job, and then the cell dies.
ACEs shorten telomeres further, leading to cells that die sooner than
they otherwise would have, and shortened telomeres are a consistent
predictor of early mortality – not just of cells but of the person who is
made of those cells.

At every level, from DNA molecules to cells, from biological systems
that regulate immunity to those that regulate pain and pleasure, from life
choices that range from whether or not to smoke to whom to sleep with,
childhood adversity tips the balance toward disease and early death.

JON IS TELLING ME about a referral he received. "The oncologist was *so*
apologetic when she asked me to see Marlene. She said 'I don't know if
Marlene will keep the appointment. If she comes, she is usually late, and
she doesn't say much. I'm not sure she really understands why she needs
treatment. That's why I'm asking you to see her. When we staged her, it
was clear that her cancer had already spread to her spine. I don't know
how she could've waited this long to come in, there is basically no breast
left – the tumor has replaced it and even broken through the skin.'"

"Yikes. Hard to imagine."

"Yeah, I know," Jon continued. "I couldn't tell from that story if Marlene was psychotic or developmentally delayed or maybe addicted to
something. Anything seemed possible; whatever it was, it was bad. So, I
dropped in to the cancer clinic when she was already there rather than
asking her to come see me separately."

Many clinicians go to see patients in clinic – the social worker, nutri-
tionist, clinical study nurses – so it feels like it's not a real psychiatry visit,
which gets the relationship off to an easier start.

"Marlene turned out to be this tiny woman wearing *layers* of cloth-ing – I don't know how many – and on top a thick cardigan, even though it wasn't cold that day. She looked like a beaten dog, honestly, shrunken back in the chair that was pushed back against the wall. The nurse knows me and gave me a big hello, which probably helped set a tone as I came in. I sat down, basically as far away from her as I could, so she wouldn't feel trapped. I told her who I was and we started talking – pretty gingerly really.

"I often frame psychiatry as just part of the normal process in the clinic. We have lots of teams and I'm part of the 'coping team,' so the Marlenes of the world don't feel singled out. I try hard not to convey, like, 'hey everybody, the shrink is here!'

"Anyway, here I was trying so hard to make sure I didn't trigger a psy-chotic thought or something, and then it turned out she wasn't psychotic or confused in the slightest. She wasn't drunk or high. She was just com-pletely freaked out. She was terrified.

"When I see someone *that* frightened, my only goal is to not make it worse so that she will be willing to see me again. Over time, we can usually build trust, but at the first meeting, it's enough to just be not part of the problem. I wanted to come across as open and accepting. Harmless. But Marlene wasn't really taking me in at all, she just wanted to get the hell out of there. She was going to say whatever would get her gone. I could see why the oncologist wasn't sure about her informed consent. Marlene just agreed with everything to get home as quickly as possible."

Jon paused. I could see that Marlene had made an impact on him.

"Over a couple of years, I met with her on clinic days, and we came to understand each other. A volunteer from her synagogue brought her to and from chemotherapy. She still lived in the house where she grew up. She had never lived anywhere else. She had nursed her parents as they aged and declined until she was the last person standing. She had a gov-ernment job that allowed her to do essentially the same task, by rote, over and over again, with little need to speak with others. It felt safe, which mattered to her more than promotion or challenge.

"Marlene's parents had both survived the Holocaust. They were so burdened by their traumas and losses that they were essentially always in their past in their heads and were absent for her. So even though she had both parents, nobody 'had' her – Marlene grew up alone."

"Like no one had her back?"

"No one had her *in mind*," Jon corrected. "She wasn't abused. No one hit her. She had clean clothes and food. But, for instance, they never got around to a Bat Mitzvah. In the absence of validation and protection, she found the world a very scary place. She went to synagogue and to work, but she hadn't had any kind of support to develop the tools to negotiate anything else.

"Living in that very small and safe routine worked well enough until Marlene felt a lump in her breast. She spent the first year convincing herself that it was nothing, that it would be gone in the morning. Planning a visit to her doctor took another year. Her doctor had scared her once, reacting with incredulity when she learned that Marlene had never had a Pap smear. Marlene felt ashamed, understanding that somehow she was a bad patient, and resolved not to go back. Now, a problem with a breast felt too personal, too sexual. Eventually, when she couldn't manage the back pain anymore, she went to Emergency instead of her family doctor because she felt less ashamed talking to a stranger."

Marlene's fear had delayed treatment by over two years. A potentially curable disease had become fatal during that time. She died from her breast cancer, eventually opting for hospice care, where people did keep her needs in mind, and eased both her pain and her loneliness. Her story is an extreme example of yet another way in which childhood adversity contributes to disease, illness, and mortality – it interferes with getting care. Growing up in scary circumstances makes it much more likely that health care will feel threatening as well. Similar things also happen in less extreme circumstances. If adversity has led a person to cope by distraction or denial, it will make it hard for them to pay attention to risks and so preventive care will suffer. If interactions with health care providers are unpleasant, it is easiest to avoid them – notice how this happens in such different ways for Isaac, who is usually angry, and for Marlene, who was always scared and prone to shame, although the consequences may be similar. If experience has taught a person not to trust authorities, they are less likely to adhere to instructions. Importantly, health care providers may not even be considered reliable sources of knowledge – a particularly harmful form of mistrust. We will see in the next chapter that even the fundamental task of telling one's health story to get help can be undermined by early adversity.

There are so many lines of dominoes in this cascade of risk that it should be no surprise that childhood adversity makes people sick and then makes it hard for them to get better. ACEs kill. They may well be one of the largest public health threats of our time. What is more surprising is that this is not more widely known, that we haven't mobilized to change it. As a society, we may be at the point now that we were in the early 1960s with respect to tobacco. The evidence is in; we know what we are dealing with; we know the challenge is huge. We're just not doing much about it.

8

"Speak for me"

The events of Isaac's childhood abuse usually followed the same pattern. The young man next door would grab Isaac as he walked between their houses and pull him into his house and down the basement stairs. What happened next became as predictable as it was terrifying.

This session, as we talked about what happened, I referred to Isaac being abducted. I wasn't trying to make a point, just referring to what happened, but the word *abducted* confused him.

"What are you talking about? I wasn't abducted."

I answer with my eyebrows and then with words. "I mean you were taken by force and held in his place against your will."

He could see that I was describing an abduction, but it still perplexed him. He just couldn't make sense of it, so we left it at that.

The next session, Isaac was off in a different direction, preoccupied by a recent event. His son, Abe, was starting his first year at university. Rooms in the dorms were in short supply. He had lost out in the lottery and was assigned to an inferior building in a sketchy area downtown, a few blocks from campus. Abe was upset, and Isaac set about fixing the situation.

Assigning kids to spots in residence is the responsibility of someone well below the dean, but Isaac didn't waste time. He phoned relentlessly until the dean agreed to see him. Once in the dean's office, Isaac made his case. When the dean started to explain the university's situation and the options that were available, Isaac interrupted him

"You think your problem is that a kid doesn't like his residence. But that's not it. Your problem is that I am in your office." He sat back, allowing his ambiguous threat to fill the room. "*I'm* your problem now."

He kept talking for a while, not letting the dean get a word in, and then he pointed down to an envelope on the desk. "I think you dropped something." Abe was assigned a new room.

I don't know if this story is true. It sounded like too much bravado to be real when I heard it. But the street-fighting one-two punch of a threat followed by a bribe is pure Isaac, the negotiator, the fixer.

In the context of our conversation, the point of the story is not his bravado though; it is the tenacity and effectiveness of his protective instinct. As a parent, Isaac is the opposite of his parents. He is a ferocious protector.

We meet the following week: "I am going to adopt a Chinese orphan."

"Where did that idea come from?"

"I've been thinking about it. I'm going to go to China and bring home an orphan and raise them like my own kids."

"What does Sarah think about that?"

"We haven't talked about it. She'll hate the idea."

I was starting to get the sense this wasn't actually a plan. It was a wild idea. Better to treat it like a thought experiment. So, I leaned in. "Why do you want to do that?"

"It's going to be an abduction. I'll take a kid away from everything it has ever known and put it in a completely foreign world where it has no choice but to stay with me. But it will be the opposite of my abduction. I'll make its world perfect. The kid will love that it has been abducted."

It wasn't a plan; it was a fantasy. Isaac was accepting the word *abduction* as it applied to him, and then turning it on its head, as if he could use his adult power to undo the damage of his own abduction. Still, the kid was an "it"; Isaac wasn't really thinking about the experience of the actual human he was rescuing, or even why the child needed his protection, but it was a rescue plan nonetheless.

I couldn't predict where we were going to go from one session to the next; I could only spot the patterns in retrospect. A week later, as we came to the end of a session, Isaac paused and then spoke.

"When you said 'abduction' it really threw me, but I think it's right. Do you know the story of Moses and Aaron?"

"I don't."

"They were brothers. God told Moses that he had to lead the Jews to the Holy Land. Moses had a speech impediment so when he had to speak to the pharaoh, Aaron spoke for him. In the end, Moses didn't make it to the Holy Land, but Aaron did."

"What are you telling me with that story?"

"I'm not going to make it. I need you to speak for me."

At the time, I thought Isaac meant that he needed me to help him find words, like *abduction*, to describe his experiences. Since then, I have realized that he also meant that he wants me to represent him to the world. Isaac is never going to tell his story to anyone but me. But he wants it to be told.

Our meetings in that couple of weeks sum up a lot of what makes Isaac such a complicated, impressive man: his formidable and sometimes intimidating strength; his determination to protect his children so that they experience none of the exploitation and neglect that he did; his bravado and wild ideas; his perplexity when he tries to understand his trauma; his hopelessness; the value he finds in our relationship.

I'm trying to live up to my part. I do think Isaac is going to make it. But I take seriously the responsibility to speak for him.

ISAAC ASKED ME, "What are you talking about?" Usually it is me wondering that about a patient.

Most meetings with patients start the same way: one person tries to tell a story and the other tries to understand it. If the meeting takes place in an Emergency Department and the storyteller is bleeding, this part of the interaction may be brief, but everything still starts there. Usually, the telling takes much longer. A great deal of what follows, the testing and the diagnosing and the treating, depends on how the first part goes. So here is something else Jon and I didn't learn in medical school: good storytellers get better care; good listeners provide better care.

Imagine you are the patient. The story you need to tell is a special one. It is the true story of what you have noticed so far about something that seems to be wrong. It is not an easy story to tell. For one thing it may feel like the stakes are high: the lump might be cancer; the pain might be untreatable. On top of that, you and I speak a different language; I have no idea what you mean by "a spell" or "woozy"; you are not relieved when I tell you the test was "negative." You rush because you appreciate my time is limited. You don't know which parts of the story are most important to me. I am listening for clues to patterns that I recognize (Does the pain wake you in the night? Does the lump hurt? Is the weakness on both sides or just one? Which symptoms are new and which are long-standing?). You may have other things to convey (you are or are not worried; you are only here because someone else said you should come; you think you know what is causing this). The conversation is challenging for each of us.

We need to help each other out with this. I listen for a while, then ask some questions because I am getting lost, or to help you to describe the patterns I am listening for, then listen some more. I need to tell you what I am thinking so you can correct the parts I am getting wrong and so that you will know when I understand. We start to adjust to each other's rhythms: now it is my turn to talk, now yours. If it goes well, it won't feel like I am applying years of training and experience to the challenge of listening well, but I am. Circumstances have made you a storyteller. My job is to make you an excellent one.

"Listen to the patient, he is telling you the diagnosis," said Dr. William Osler. Physicians still need the advice. A classic study found that when doctors speak with patients, on average they interrupt them in about eighteen seconds. A much more recent study has updated this finding for the modern era. As physicians, we have progressed; we have our interrupting time down to eleven seconds now. Communication skills are an essential part of the curriculum for future health care providers, but we obviously still have work to do, and the unrecognized effects of childhood adversity raise the stakes.

Of all the ways that childhood adversity makes people sick and then makes it hard for them to get better, perhaps the least recognized is that early adversity plays havoc with storytelling skills. Trauma leads to *narrative incoherence*. I see it often with Isaac. It doesn't matter that he is intelligent and articulate; it isn't about that. His defenses against appreciating his traumatic memories interfere with sensemaking. This form of incoherence manifests as incomprehension: "What are you talking about? I wasn't abducted." Or the dozens of times he has asked, "What happened to me?" It is a plain question, not rhetorical, not metaphorical, and it leads to weird conversations in which I tell him what happened to him (which I have learned from him) only to find that it makes no sense; the facts seem to miss the point. This is incoherence resulting from a brain not working right, or as Isaac puts it, from being a brain that is "fucked up beyond repair." I hope he is overstating the permanence of the problem.

Narrative incoherence also manifests as a misunderstanding about the *purpose* of communication. This happens when I assume that Isaac speaks to be understood, to convey some information, when in fact he speaks to feel safe. When Isaac tells me in Chapter 3, "I could be a terrorist ... I could do that," his goal is to be the strongest guy in the room, no matter what room he is in, to be invincible. I can hear his declaration as a statement of advocacy for the oppressed, like the oppressed little boy he was, but he would not agree. He would insist, I think, that I take him literally. Even if I were to appreciate that he needs to be intimidating to feel safe and try the psychotherapy trick of translating his statement into that underlying message ("I wonder if you are saying that to intimidate, to make sure that no one can mess with you"), I think he might still insist on a literal reading – because my trick would render his words into a communication of his inner state, and the point is that their intent is to keep his inner state safe, which means private.

Sometimes, people who maintain their safety and security by keeping emotional distance from others, as Isaac does, use a kind of pseudo-communication that allows them to participate in a conversation without giving much away. Often, they provide conclusions without evidence or elaboration. For example, "What was your dad like?" "Oh, he was a good guy. Brought home the bacon." Being provided with a conclusion tends to shut a conversation down. It does not invite further inquiry. This example is also typical in its use of clichés, which leave the listener to fill in their own meaning.

In a medical setting, when a health care provider is asking questions to understand a problem, this style of communicating leads to a short and unilluminating conversation. If I ask how something painful feels, for example, none of these answers advance the diagnostic process much: "It's bad," "It's not too bad," "How do you think it feels?" "Just help me get this back under control." Communication that is the opposite of collaboration uses generalizations without examples, conclusions without evidence, statements without elaboration, and commands without context. Their point is to maintain distance.

Master storytellers read their audience. They see which jokes are working, how long to leave a pause, when to add emphasis. The process is collaborative. Technically, when the story's audience is just one person, this is called *mentalizing*: the storytellers are forming and testing hypotheses about what is in their audience's mind as they spin the tale. A person like Isaac, when talking to a doctor or nurse about something that makes him feel unwell, is not mentalizing. He is not wondering what this person needs to know to help him or how well they are understanding him at a particular moment. He is in a conversation that feels dangerous. He doesn't expect it to go well. A good outcome would be that this person figures out on their own what will help and does it. He wouldn't be here if he felt he had any other choice. Most other outcomes include disappointment, pain, humiliation, or conflict. He has neither the wish nor the capacity to tell his story well in this moment, and his medical care suffers for it.

So, one pattern of communication that follows from early adversity is to distance or contain things, like Isaac does. His defenses place a wall between him and those who can harm him. Unfortunately, they also place a wall between him and those who could provide solace. His pattern is sometimes called *dismissing*, because it is dismissing of the need to trust and rely on others.

The other main pattern is the opposite: uncontained communication that has no walls or structure. This pattern is just as bad for telling the story of one's health, maybe worse. People with this pattern are too overwhelmed by fear to organize their thoughts. Events are out of sequence, gradations of severity are lost because everything is really bad. There are no storytelling clues about which bits are the important parts, and characters appear without introduction. It is like the story of this person's health was made into a jigsaw puzzle, and all the pieces were dumped on the table at once – except that it isn't a puzzle we can noodle over; it is urgent. This style of communicating conveys the source of a problem very poorly but the need for urgent help very effectively. If Isaac's communication pushes a listener away, this pattern pulls a listener in – making them an essential partner in constructing the story, a prosthetic organizer of events, sensations, and reactions. This pattern is simply called *anxious*, or more technically, *preoccupied*, because the person is preoccupied with distress and with their need to stay close to someone who can help.

It is my job to help people tell their story well. All of the biological marvels of modern medical treatment have to wait until we finish that part. Before I can prescribe wonder-mycin and panacea-cillin, I need to know what we are treating.

Think how this applies to the many adults who have experienced substantial childhood adversity, the more than nine million Canadians and sixty million Americans whose health care is compromised by the consequences of fear, which interfere with telling their story well enough to get the best care. ACEs do not just cause disease and illness; they render illness indistinct and puzzling. They force health care providers to confront their limited skills as interpreters of stories and collaborators in communication, roles that many health care providers don't even *want*, let alone are skilled in. They render the magnificent achievements of biological medicine irrelevant, at least for a while, as we try to piece together what is going on. A patient and I can't begin to use most of the tools of medicine until we have used its most fundamental tool – our relationship – to secure a base from which we can do our work.

9

Fever

When we were about two years into therapy, things got weird with me. Isaac was all in, and I was in the shit with him. The complicated layers of trouble Isaac was trying to sort out were often communicated in dreams, which he was now reporting regularly.

The dreams were perverse, anatomical, frightening, and almost incoherent. They contained elements of his actual experiences and other details that would make more sense in a horror movie. Isaac would wake from these dreams and be unable to go back to sleep, afraid that someone was going to break into his house. He would get out of bed, sit in the front room, smoke a cigarette, and keep watch.

Around this point, I started to change. The initial signs were benign and ambiguous. I started to wear neckties, which was not my style at the time, though Isaac wore ties. I thought more often than usual about our conversations. I went home from work irritable and miserable. I was fighting with my wife, Lynn, blaming her for everything and feeling picked on.

And then I started to dream.

I don't usually remember my dreams. When I do, they are not very interesting. Lynn has dreams that are adventures with spies and dramatic plot lines, dreams that will be cast with top-flight Hollywood actors when they are eventually brought to the big screen. My dreams reveal the mundane worries of someone who is responsible, obsessive, and sensitive. I am late for something, there is an exam that I have not prepared for, I am laboring beneath the weight of an unclear obligation. But in the period in which I wore ties and found arguments around every corner, I had different dreams. I don't remember them all clearly, but they were perverse, anatomical, frightening, and almost incoherent.

I woke from these dreams feeling too ashamed at their content to talk about them and too troubled to ignore them. At some point I recognized that Isaac was right; his trouble is contagious. I was in it with him now, and I was in too far. Jon had told me to hang on, but I was losing my grip. I was dressing to be Isaac and to protect myself from him, as if a man in an open collar might be overpowered by a man with a necktie. The conflict I was finding in my most important relationship, with Lynn, was actually coming from within me. I was both the aggressor and the victim. And I was having Isaac's dreams.

Many years earlier, I went through four years of psychoanalysis as part of my training. I sometimes joke that although I finished the analysis, it didn't take. It's only half a joke. The dreams made me realize that it was time for a top-up. I approached a colleague who I knew was good and whose discretion I trusted and asked him to see me for therapy. When I explained the situation, he asked if I wanted supervision rather than therapy – someone to watch over my work as a therapist and give me advice. I said no. Working with Isaac demanded spontaneity; I felt like I had to be nimble. I couldn't do it well if I felt like I had a supervisor looking over my shoulder. I needed a therapist.

So my colleague and I met for a few months. I talked about Isaac a lot and about myself, about Lynn and my family and parents a bit, and we sorted things out. I went back to dressing the way I like, I went back to my boring familiar dreams, and I stopped picking fights. It didn't make the work that Isaac and I were doing any easier. But I could at least leave most of it in my office when I went home.

My reaction was more intense and sustained than usually happens for psychotherapists. Nonetheless, it is not unusual for therapists to be strongly affected by emotions that emerge from listening to their patients with empathy. Those who have not experienced it may be surprised.

A mentor of mine, who is far better at psychotherapy than I will ever be, talks about the emotional temperature that a therapist should maintain when being affected by a patient: hot enough to be engaged, but cool enough to think. By that criteria, in 2000, I had a fever. Having succeeded in cooling down since then, I don't regret that I am affected by Isaac's story. I accept that you have to take at least a little damage in this work to have a small appreciation of what it feels like to be as damaged as Isaac thinks he is. I reset the thermostat and we carried on.

Sometimes you need a professional to help you be yourself. That's something else that Isaac and I have in common.

"YOU'RE IN IT WITH ME NOW." Staying hot enough to be engaged and cool enough to think is not easy. In late 2000, I had a fever, but a prolonged cold spell is more common for me and for most practitioners.

Chapter 5 described the hidden curriculum that privileges health care providers and disempowers patients, dividing the two into us and them. When in doubt about the distinction, we professionals can remind ourselves, as we learned from The House of God, that "the patient is the one with the disease." This division and the blindness of medicine to the role of childhood adversity in creating and perpetuating illness and disease seem intertwined.

To acknowledge that one in three of our patients has been seriously maltreated, and that this is a strong force in their disease and suffering, is to acknowledge the same about ourselves. One in three is too many to only apply to them. Our research backs this up. We find that childhood trauma is just as common among people who work in hospitals as it is for anyone else. Maybe a little more common, but definitely not less. For some first responders, the rates are much higher; we found that 44 per cent of female paramedics reported having experienced physical, sexual, or emotional abuse when they were girls, suggesting that having had that experience might motivate some people to seek work as a first responder.

Health care professionals have special skills, but they aren't special people; they aren't superheroes. So, if society as a whole turns a blind eye to the harms of child maltreatment, as it certainly does, then health care professionals are likely to have the same deficit. Beyond that, health care professionals, as normally functioning human beings, have to do *something* to not feel so bad about all of the sad crap they deal with – the suffering, the dying, and the uselessness of so much of our effort. Not to mention the barriers to doing things that might work – the hours wasted on poorly designed electronic medical records or the insurers who refuse to pay for treatment. We do what all humans do to cope. We distance, laugh, blame, objectify, and deny, and less often appreciate, join, listen, acknowledge, and cry. Since this is what we do to cope with the trouble that comes from working in health care, it only makes sense that as a group we would apply the same strategies to defend ourselves against the role of childhood maltreatment in our work. Maybe it should not be surprising that Jon and I took a few years working in our field to realize that so many of our patients were dealing with the consequences of childhood adversity.

Unfortunately, these defenses do not fully protect health care professionals. They may even perpetuate the pain – suppressed truths, secrets that humans keep from even themselves, tend to fuel suffering. Interpersonal distance is generally unhealthy. Inflexible divisions between us and them also seem an unlikely recipe for healing. Further, health care has high occupational risks. Nurses are exposed to physical and emotional abuse alarmingly frequently. Suicide rates are elevated in female physicians and in some specialties, such as psychiatry and anesthesia. Burnout, which includes feeling emotionally exhausted, treating patients like objects, and losing any sense of professional accomplishment, is rampant, affecting between a quarter and a third of health care professionals. Not surprisingly, burned-out providers provide poor care; they make more mistakes, and their patients are less safe. Indeed, burnout about doubles the odds that a physician will be involved in a "patient safety incident."

Most of medicine does not demand as much tolerance of intimacy and close listening as psychotherapy does. It makes more sense to speak of staying open and listening well then of staying "hot enough to be engaged," but the basic setup is the same for all health care professionals. The attitudes that are required to bring down the wall that separates us and them are not complex: curiosity, respect, and attention to cues that indicate that a person has something to say.

Health care providers also need to manage two dueling truths. They are self-evident and yet stand in opposition to each other. The first is that everyone is different: you can't know someone's experience without asking; you can't assume; you need an open mind. The second is that we are all the same: we are all insecure; we do whatever we need to do to find safety, comfort, and love.

One very specific and pertinent example of health care professionals being open to their patients' experience is asking adult patients about childhood adversity. It doesn't happen very often. Surveys and interviews of patients and of doctors seem to agree on the current state of affairs. Patients understand that the question is relevant and don't mind being asked as long as it is done in a way that feels safe and respectful, but they are not likely to volunteer a story of maltreatment unless invited. Some doctors, particularly the younger ones, appreciate that they should ask, but mostly don't. A survey of doctors that we conducted suggested their behavior depends on their specialty. Psychiatrists usually ask about childhood adversity; other specialists rarely do. Most family doctors said that they ask patients about childhood adversity when they think it "is indicated" to do so. Family doctors tell us that this isn't very often. Outside of psychiatry, it is not a standard part of an initial assessment.

Why would that be? Patients who have spoken about being asked about childhood adversity usually favor the idea, so it appears that the resistance is mostly on the side of the doctors. For their part, doctors have reasons not to ask. Most say they don't have enough time, although it only takes a few minutes. They don't know what to do with the answer. Specialists assume that the information is irrelevant to their practice, which is not the case. Our survey suggested that physicians who know that childhood adversity is linked to *physical* diseases were more likely to ask about it, so awareness may help.

We suspect that the biggest barrier is doctors' discomfort. Many doctors, especially specialists, don't tolerate sitting with suffering that they cannot fix (oddly, since that is our main business). They believe that a positive answer to a question about childhood adversity would cause distress and require referring their patient to mental health specialists, who are in short supply. Evidence suggests that *just asking* doesn't create brand new needs for mental health care. The information is new *to you*, dear doctor, not to the patient who is telling you about it. It does not become an emergency because you asked. It becomes *shared*.

And what is the value of that? Sharing a critically important, emotionally complex piece of a person's story changes the nature of your relationship. You have been entrusted with something valuable. You don't know if it is also fragile. You need to demonstrate that you are worthy of trust, that you are thoughtful and listening. Although it won't be part of the conversation, the information may reverberate with your own experiences or with those of someone you love. One in three people have suffered from serious adversity, whether or not they have medical degrees.

That is what doctors resist, I think. Although the conversation will only be of one person's experience, while the other listens, learns, and tries to understand, it is not the interrogation of *them* by *us* that is troubling; it is the sharing. The thing that is shared happened long ago; it cannot be fixed. If the experience causes suffering (it doesn't always; you can't assume; you need to listen), then it is the kind of suffering that may be hard to treat. This is the kind of conversation that can build a relationship in which healing is a possibility, one of trust and safety, one that acknowledges what patients and health care providers have in common – that we are all doing our best to face suffering that we can't fix and to help each other. As it happens, this is a special conversation because one partner in it has special skills and access to the vault of science, but it is built on shared humanity. Sharing stories, which in this context mostly means listening intently and trying to understand, is revolutionary.

A career in health care has occupational risks. Ironically, building walls against those risks may contribute to them. I paid the price for letting down the wall and getting too close to Isaac's contagious memories of terror. Now, with my defenses snapped back into place, I try to help my colleagues to peek over the top.

10

Partialists

Crohn's disease is miserable. It causes pernicious fatigue, fever, painful joints, gut pain, diarrhea, and loss of appetite, with one kind of suffering alternating with the next unpredictably. It is hard for people who don't have it to appreciate what it is like. The best we can do is to think of our own illnesses that came and went. But those transient ailments miss key parts of living with Crohn's disease, which are its perpetuity and the constant threat that something worse is about to happen. You are either sick or about to be.

At the time of this story, something worse was emerging out of the constant shift of Isaac's symptoms. He was having bowel obstructions every few weeks and the frequency was increasing. They are a sign that the gut has reached a critical limit. The tissues that form the wall of the intestine, which is really just a hose, have become so swollen with inflammation that nothing can pass through the center. With luck and care, the swelling will go down after a few hours of excruciating pain and the system will restart. If not, surgery.

Isaac knew from painful experience that at some point, he would arrive at the obstruction that doesn't clear, the one that requires emergency surgery. In spite of the detached arithmetic about surgical bowel resections that Isaac had presented to me when we first met, he was wary of another operation. He went to see a surgeon for an opinion – would it be wiser to have the surgery now or to roll the dice on the chance that the obstructions would subside? The surgeon's answer was cautious, but she was leaning toward acting now.

Back in my office, the fearful expectations that had been burned into Isaac's brain by childhood trauma kicked in.

"I read about this guy who woke up while they were doing surgery on him. They didn't know it but he was aware of the whole thing. He was paralyzed, but he was awake."

"It's pretty rare, but it happens. You're thinking of your own surgery?"

"It's going to happen to me. They'll be cutting my stomach open. Cutting out my intestine. Sewing me. And I'm going to be awake, like I'm watching it and feeling it."

My lips pursed a bit, conveying my skepticism. "It's rare, so probably not. And if it happened, they would figure it out and fix it."

"No, it's going to happen. They'll be oblivious."

"You're scared of what happens when you aren't able to protect yourself?"

"I can't stand the idea of being unconscious with people inside me. I can't do that again. Going unconscious."

"So both options, being conscious and being unconscious in surgery, are terrifying."

"Yeah. My only option is not to do it."

"But you may not have an option, the way the obstructions are going."

"I always have an option." Suicide was Isaac's trump card.

I leaned back in my chair, resigning the point. "Okay."

Isaac paused and took a different tack. "After the surgery, you get morphine. That's fantastic. But you should get as much as you want. I'll never accept my pain being under someone else's control."

"Has the pain control not been enough after your other operations?"

"I just lie in the bed and it really hurts and they decide how much I should hurt. Fuck that. Why shouldn't I have the drugs?"

"I know. How much pain medication is the right amount can be a point of contention after surgery."

I regretted the phrase "can be a point of contention" as soon as it came out of my mouth. It was a sign that, once again, the obligations of my profession were screwing up my empathy. It is hard for a doctor to empathize with Isaac when he is endorsing suicide and addiction. If it is hard for me when I have empathy as my primary goal, it must be near-impossible for surgeons and other specialists who have other goals.

"I should have as much as I want."

"They want to treat your pain well, but they don't want to give you more than you need and cause more problems."

"They don't give a shit about my pain. They just do what they want."

Isaac was at risk of putting off surgery that would be much easier to recover from if he had it in a planned way before it became an emergency. There were rational arguments to wait and see how things went for a while, but those were not the arguments that were guiding him. He was guided by the expectation that his suffering would be ignored and that others would control him without regard to his well-being or wishes. And he was guided by his intolerance of the idea of giving up all control to trust others (in his case, a series of others – a gastroenterologist, a surgeon, an anesthetist, nurses, and their students), which is the basic contract of a patient having surgery.

You might think that having gone through it before would make it easier or at least that Isaac had made his peace with repeated operations by now. His bravado on the first day we met would suggest so. But fear doesn't always answer to logic. And repeating a trauma doesn't make it easier the next time. Combat soldiers know that. It doesn't get easier as you go. It gets worse. Same for Isaac.

Childhood trauma can affect virtually all aspects of the choices that people make about health care, but it is rarely as explicit and as dramatic as it is when Isaac needs another operation.

JON WALKS INTO MY OFFICE for our Monday meeting waving a few faxed pages at me. He had picked up his mail on the way.

"Look at this!" he says. "This is why we need to write this book. Un-fucking-believable."

"What?" I had no idea what he was talking about.

"My patient, Charlotte, wasn't getting better. So I needed a fresh set of eyes and I asked for a second opinion from Don, because he's been in the business for a long time."

He went on without pausing. "I first saw Charlotte when she was adjusting to having a mastectomy for breast cancer. Over time it became clear that her problems hadn't started with cancer. That was just when things piled up on her, and there was a relatively easy route to psychiatry via the cancer clinic. Turns out she had been seriously depressed for years, mostly because of crap she had endured in her early years. She doesn't remember her father, because he died when she was four, but he sounds like a bit of an asshole. Anyway, her mother had fallen apart afterward, spending her days in a dark room. Charlotte remembered coming home from school not knowing what she would find. Sometimes her mother, passed out drunk. Sometimes an empty house. When Charlotte was twelve, her mother remarried and then directed most of her attention to her new partner, Murray. Charlotte prefers not to talk about Murray but called him 'handsy.'

"Charlotte excelled at school and played on every sports team so she could stay away from home as long as possible. School was so much better than home. She was self-reliant to a fault. Essentially, she raised herself. But her self-esteem was based on achievements, people praising her for getting that big goal. That is hard to sustain, and doesn't always happen. Most of us aren't the star player. Of course, with no one conveying that *she* counted – as opposed to her *achievements* – Charlotte doubted that she was really worthy of praise, even when she got it. Later on, closer to the time she came to me, her marriage hit the rocks and then she got cancer. Her life basically collapsed – she was back living on her own, trying to stay occupied – like staying late at school again – but became too sick and tired to manage that, so she was left with all the old baggage just banging around inside her head but now keeping company with fears of death and disability. She tried to be a good patient like she had been a good athlete and became a relentlessly positive thinker, because that's what the world was telling her she had to be: a 'star' patient. But it took tons of effort because she had never had the sense that things would end well. On her own, out of the public eye, she felt seriously crappy. The effort to be positive was exhausting her even more than the treatment was.

"I met with her in psychotherapy to see if she could find a way of feeling okay about herself that wasn't so fragile and effortful. For her meds, I followed the treatment guidelines. But it wasn't really helping, so I figured it was time for advice from someone else, who might see a new angle that I wasn't seeing. So I called Don."

"I got the letter back just now ... Six pages! ... Don's got Charlotte's whole story, from the details of her symptoms, through the family history of psychiatric illnesses and the prior treatment trials, to the adversity she experienced growing up. *He got the whole fucking story!* Obviously, he spent the time required to appreciate it all. And then, he suggests Effexor. And if that doesn't work ... wait for it ... 'consider adding lithium.'"

Jon sat up straight, the way he does when he is passionate about a topic, and spoke very deliberately. "There is not a goddamn word in any of his treatment recommendations about Charlotte's life and no attempt to put her depression into context. Even though he spoke to her about her life, there is no signal that he had it in mind when trying to suggest what to do. It's like he saw talking as a means of getting a good interview, but then discarded it when he started thinking about what to do, like the only kind of treatment he could consider was meds. You know I'd be delighted to try a new med, and will follow his advice, but Don knows as well as I do that by the time you've tried two or three, there is a diminishing return, so I was hoping for, you know, *reflective feedback*. Why bother talking first, if all you're going to do is categorize her diagnosis, and then push 'play' on the textbook advice? I don't know what I was hoping for, but this sure as shit ain't it." He slumped back in his chair. I didn't say anything.

Most doctors are partialists. That is what our colleague, Ross Upshur, an expert in the actual complexity of living with and treating chronic medical conditions, renames specialists. We only treat our bits. If some-one has a problem that extends outside our narrow purview, we don't stretch to say, "I think this might be a-certain-something-or-other that is outside of my expertise. Let me put you in touch with someone who is excellent with that. I'll see you again too in case I am wrong," or "I can help you with a part of that, but I think you're going to need a team," or "Let's step back here and try to understand the big picture." In the worst case, we just say, "Nah, that doesn't look like what I treat. Next!"

When Charlotte met Don, he provided exactly the suggestions that one would expect from a partialist. His six-page, comprehensive letter and evidence-based medication advice surpassed the usual standard of care. But he didn't do Charlotte much good. We need more doctors who are working to pay attention to the whole person in front of them.

Aside from his family doctor, Simon, who tries to hold it all together, Isaac navigates between partialists who are spaced like islands in the roil-ing ocean of his illness. Maybe the next one will bring relief and a safe harbor. But, to push the metaphor a bit too far, communication between the island nations is dismal and customs control is slow and arbitrary. It is easy for him to believe that "they don't give a shit about my pain. They just do what they want." It is a miserable setup for someone who was trained from a young age to mistrust authority and offers of care. There is little in this system, when it operates as usual, that would help Isaac overcome his dramatic, bizarre fears of surgery, for example. The system makes it easy for him to believe that the only course that will allow him to have control over his body and his health is to maintain his option for suicide.

11

"What are we doing here?"

"What happened to me?"

Each time Isaac asks this question, and he has asked this many times over the years, is like the first. He is like someone with a concussion after a head injury who doesn't realize that he is asking the same perplexed, anguished question for the twentieth time. Not quite like that because he does know that he has asked before, but that is the impression he creates.

Since it is clear from previous conversations that he means, "What happened to me when I was ten?" I try to answer.

I hold my hands out slightly, bringing us the tiniest bit closer together. "You were harmed. It wasn't your fault. You were overpowered and terrified. It stayed a secret for a long time. You eventually got away but you weren't rescued."

"But what happened to me?"

"Do you mean what did that experience do to you?"

"I don't know."

My answers to these questions always baffle Isaac. That is weird because the only reason that I have any answers is that he has told me what happened in other conversations. He knows but he doesn't know. Isaac is a man whose power of logic and argument is so strong that he can be intimidating. As a union official, he wins arguments for a living. And yet in these moments he is uncomprehending and all-but-incomprehensible.

Probably because of fear, trauma leaves holes in a person's ability to understand and communicate. I had a colleague who once sent me an unusually long and convoluted email about being away for the afternoon to visit the dentist. At the bottom, having recognized that his complicated message didn't make sense, he wrote "dental phobia, therefore gibberish." In a moment of fear, anyone can become incoherent.

Forgetting is one way to protect oneself from memories that trigger terror or shame. Or things get disconnected, memories are stored and retrieved unconnected to the emotions that would usually accompany them. Or sense-making fails, as it did when Isaac couldn't understand how I could call his experience an abduction. In each case, the distortions make it harder to tell a coherent story about one's life. Completely overwhelming experiences are so confusing and unintelligible that they probably prevent clear memories from being made in the first place.

The explanation that resonates for Isaac is that his brain is broken. He says that his brain is completely fucked up. Isaac, the persuader and negotiator, has big gaps in his otherwise powerful intellect.

The perplexed and child-like state that is communicated by the question "What happened to me?" would not be an issue for his physical health except that one of the triggers of this incoherence is pain. The phrase that Isaac remembers most clearly from his experiences of abuse, probably never spoken aloud at the time but repeated in his head a thousand times, is "this is going to hurt." The anticipation that "this is going to hurt" continues to be a potent trigger of his least coherent form of thinking. What he says becomes ambiguous. His expectation that he will be hurt is so strongly connected to memories of how he was hurt in the past that it overwhelms his ability to assess what is actually going on in the present. He looks wild and scary in those moments. For health care that works best when communication supports collaboration, Isaac's expectation that he is going to be hurt is a setup for inferior care.

Unfortunately, he has a disease that hurts, that requires tests that hurt and sometimes treatments that hurt. Of course, it doesn't go well.

"What are we doing here?"

I look Isaac in the eye and try to read what is behind his question. I can't tell, but I am pretty sure he is waiting for a response. "I'm going to answer that. It is an ambiguous question so my answer may not match what you intend, but I'll try. We are having a conversation to try to change how you think and feel and how you remember traumatic things. We are doing it because it seems to help."

"Yeah, but what are we doing?"

"I'm going to take that to mean 'why does it help?'" Isaac nods a bit.

"I don't know for sure, but I think there are a few things going on. One is that you say things out loud that you usually keep silent about, and I try to listen well. I think saying things out loud changes them. Another is that I think that we, I mean people, remember traumatic things in very different ways from usual memories. So, when you and I talk about these things, we complicate them, and connect them to other memories and ideas, and join them up with normal memories. I think that makes those bad memories a little more 'normal,' which allows you to deal with them differently, even if they still feel just as bad. And also, I work hard to earn your trust. That is a different kind of relationship for you and I think that makes a difference." I realize as I am speaking that I have been counting these three things off on my fingers. It is unusual for me to offer Isaac an opinion that might sound authoritative and my body has slipped into gestures that I use when teaching.

Isaac picks up on talking about how memory works. "There are these memory prodigies who remember way more than most people. One of these guys says he takes all the things he is trying to remember and puts them in certain places in this big house he has in his mind."

"There are different tricks like that," I respond. "I don't think it matters much what you are connecting the memories to, whatever works for you. It is the extra connections that help."

"I think you could do it with music. I don't know how, but I think you could." Isaac sat silently for a minute or two. "When I am around my nephew's kid, I am so worried that something bad is going to happen to him. That someone is going to do something. I don't want my nephew to take him on vacation because I am so worried something is going to happen. I mean crazy worried. It's way over the top. I try not to say everything I'm thinking. I would sound crazy."

"So, that's what I mean. That counts as progress with what we're doing. You're thinking on two tracks. One is the crazy intense worry that something is going to happen to your nephew's kid, like it happened to you. But you are not just re-experiencing that fear, you are also observing it. There is another part of your mind on another track, going, 'That's way over the top. I better try to control that. The world is not as dangerous for my nephew's kid as it feels to me.'"

"Yeah, I know." Isaac averted his eyes.

The work that Isaac and I do together helps him tell better stories. It helps him observe himself with a clearer mind. When he has others in his mind, he imagines what they may be thinking or feeling a little more accurately.

Our conversation is working, I guess. Isaac has a good relationship with his family doctor now. He finally found a gastroenterologist who listens and whom he trusts. He can go to the Emergency Department if he has to, and sometimes it helps.

PSYCHOTHERAPY IS LIKE PARENTING in some ways. The comparison is not meant to diminish or infantilize patients, or to exaggerate the role that therapists have in their patients' lives, which can be modest, but merely to notice that there are a few similarities. Like parents and their children, it is not an equal or reciprocal relationship – the two of you have different roles, abilities, and power. A therapist is also like a parent because they are really trying to make the relationship work for the benefit of the other. And it is very complicated. You can't know what you are doing all the time. Therapy can last a long time, so therapists can't possibly be at their best all the time. With Isaac, I follow some principles, but I also make well-intentioned guesses along the way. That is not so different from my experience as a parent.

"Parents who read this book are going to be a bit freaked out, I think," Jon said as we sat down for a Monday meeting.

"I can think of some reactions," I agreed. "Some will think that the story of ACEs is another 'blame the parents' or especially 'blame the mothers' sort of theory, which will either scare them or piss them off or both."

"No shit. Of course it would if you read that as the intent."

"Others will think 'Oh my God, I've wrecked my kids! All I do is invalidate my son or daughter.'"

"That's the one I was thinking of. People will remember the last time they were tired or impatient and told their kid to stop being so annoying ... and then feel awful."

"And maybe some will look at Isaac's mom and dad and think, 'Well, they are terrible. At least I'm better than that.'"

"That's something, I guess." Jon smiled. "I think we need to talk about 'good enough' parenting. That kids don't need perfection; they just need parents who are there for them enough. Consistent enough, responsive enough, protective enough ..." He paused.

"Not only is it good enough to be good enough, but it is actually optimal," he continued. "Parents need to be there enough that kids are safe and protected and feel loved, but kids also need some space on their own for personal development, to develop self-regulation and confidence. So good enough is not a lower standard; it is an optimal balance. The balance idea makes me think of the beach in PEI," said Jon, referring to the place his family vacations every summer. "It is a big, long, flat beach with shallow tide pools. You can see the kids from way off and it's a perfect place for them to wander and explore, and go and pick up shells, or follow a hermit crab into the water or fall down in a tide pool, and they're safe - well, you know, safe *enough*. And that feeling of exploring is a good kid-feeling to have -"

I interrupt. "So, that is the idea of parenting as a kind of rubber-band connection - kids feel good and confident and curious, so they wander away, and if they get scared or hurt, they come running back and you are there to help them feel better. I love the image of your family on the beach for that idea, even though it applies everywhere, in the living room when your kid is learning to walk, in their teens when they are exploring the world or exploring new ideas."

Jon carries on. "You have two tasks as a parent. One is to stand back and let kids explore, knowing that it might be great or it might end in tears. The other is to be there ready if that happens, so they can run back into your arms until everything feels okay again, or to celebrate with them when it is a 'win.'"

"I remember when our second son was first walking," I said. "I don't remember that this was such an issue for the first, but our second – he was always running and smashing into things. He would get cuts or bruises, especially on his face, and we would feel like we had to be on high alert, but you also had to let him do his thing. It was impossible to feel you were getting it right. We couldn't really contain him, he was too determined, but then he gets another mark on the face and I'm thinking, *I'm a shit parent.*"

"And you're thinking, *All the neighbors think I'm a monster,*" adds Jon.

"Exactly."

"There are always two tasks. Always both at the same time." Jon was getting animated; his voice was probably starting to carry into the next office and he was using his hands for emphasis. "It's always keep them safe, but let them explore. Build their confidence, but let them fail. It's always both things. If you simplify parenting to just 'keep your child safe,' you squash development. If you simplify parenting to 'a child needs to explore,' they won't feel safe enough to explore. It's always both things. And to know which of those they need from you *right now,* you just need to pay attention to them 'cause they'll tell you when they need comforting and when you're crowding them. Paying attention to their cues and responding is the key to being good enough and having secure kids."

"That is 'sensitive responsiveness,'" I add. "The evidence says that the most important thing to promote security is sensitivity and responsiveness and not, say, being emotionally warm. Warmth is good, of course, but the key is responsiveness."

"Because responsiveness is a characteristic of a *relationship* ... It's about two people figuring it out. It's not just a quality of a parent; it is the parent and the kid figuring it out together."

I hesitate, putting my thoughts together. "I think that is why being good enough is the best that is available. Because you are always responding to the other person. You can't just 'be perfect,' whatever that means. You are always adjusting, reacting, missing the mark, and then recalibrating."

"It's a tennis game, you are always responding to the last shot. No, that is too competitive a metaphor. It's a dance," Jon summarizes.

"Also because the kid is always different. I mean one kid is not the same as another kid. Parents who think they have things figured out with their first kid are in for a shock when they have a second. Like when our second son started smashing into everything when he was learning to run. They are so different from one another. Also, a kid on Tuesday morning is different from the same kid on Tuesday afternoon. You are always adjusting."

"And to be real, sometimes what you are adjusting from is that you weren't paying attention for a while, or you were distracted by your own troubles, or whatever."

We pause for a second and Jon adds, "I think we should also say something about consistency. That the thing that matters most is what usually happens. One of the troubles with how ACEs are described is that it makes people think about singular events. But it isn't really particular events that usually matter. It's the overall pattern. The sorts of experiences that are repeated a thousand times ... and also, that for a lot of kids who have some ACEs but are okay as adults, there is often someone else in the story, maybe a grandparent or nanny, who was consistent and responsive, which kind of saves the day, so they are able to put the ACEs behind them."

"So, the message to parents is 'Congratulations on being imperfect. That is excellent. Pay attention to the cues your kid is giving you so that you can respond when they need you to. No matter what you do, it isn't going to be exactly right a lot of the time. That's okay. Tune back in and keep dancing.' Something like that."

Jon gets up to go. "Yeah. And ask our kids how we did. We won't get straight A's. But I think we've been good enough, often enough."

12

Gifts

For a few weeks in the second year of therapy, Isaac was bringing a new dream to discuss every time we met, sometimes several.

A ten-year-old boy with adult genitalia is masturbating. The boy is unaware that he is being observed by Isaac as an adult.

"It is completely incongruous. It is wrong. I'm a perverse, sick fuck."

The boy implodes and forms a dark projectile that gets embedded in Isaac-the-adult's abdomen.

"That is the Crohn's, the gut pain I guess," I said, "and also the painful experience of being assaulted maybe. You are the boy-you and the adult-you. In the dream, you also seem to be both the kid and the adult getting off. In the dream, you are everyone."

The observer in the dream is now ten-year-old Isaac, no longer an adult.

"You are beside me, crouched over with your arm around my shoulder. You are going to explain it to me. You're not saying, 'don't worry, it will be okay.' You're saying, 'I can help you understand this.' ... And then I am lying in bed. I think I have woken up from these sick dreams. A guy comes in with a big knife and stabs me in the back. I can see my back and this huge wound turns into a vagina."

"Even waking up is not an escape. There is too much here to understand, but we can start." The dream tells me that my role is to help Isaac understand, not to give empty reassurances, so I take that direction. "Some of these images are pretty close to your actual experience, and some are new twists. Like that you can move between being right in the memory and being an observer and that you may not have to be alone with it."

The pain in Isaac's abdomen gets worse as we talk about the dreams. His gut and his memories are often linked like this. Sometimes it gets better when we speak, but not today.

I am about to take a vacation, so the ending of the session feels a little more final than usual. Isaac stands up to leave and I stand up to see him off. His first step is toward me instead of to the door. He reaches out and offers an envelope. Our chairs are six or seven feet apart, so I take a step toward him to receive it.

"You need this to protect you," he says.

In the envelope is a penknife. A very small one, almost just a decoration, but with a real blade. The message is ambiguous. In another context it might come across as a threat, but I know that Isaac cares for me. He is trying to protect me from the harm that he thinks he has brought.

After I return from holiday, we continue to talk about the dreams, making sense of them piece by piece, as best we can.

Anyone who comes into my office knows that I like music. Up high near the ceiling, the walls are decorated with framed album covers. Some are famous (The Clash's *London Calling*, The Band's *Music from Big Pink*), some are obscure (*Got No Breeding* by Jules and the Polar Bears), and a couple are signed. On the bookshelves are Beatles knickknacks (the Russian dolls, an action figure of John from Yellow Submarine, a music box). There is a photograph of an accordion player at a kitchen party. The musical theme is obvious.

Isaac loves music too. Beyond knowing his dreams, I know that Isaac loves Elvis, especially the gospel songs. We once found out in conversation that we had read the same memoir of the musician, Warren Zevon, who is famous to a certain kind of music fan but unknown to many people. It is the kind of coincidence that can make people feel more closely connected.

As we end another session, Isaac reaches into the pocket of his suit jacket and unfolds a piece of paper. It is a list, printed off in a large font. As he hands it to me, I can see that it is a band's set list from a concert.

"I got this for you."

"Thank you. What is it?"

I looked at the set list: *Kokomo, Surfer Girl, Rhonda.*

"I saw the Beach Boys last week."

"Oh, wow."

"Yeah, it was great. I stayed after. I went backstage."

I didn't say anything, but I was impressed with his chutzpah. I would never try to go backstage at a concert, but I could imagine Isaac pulling it off.

"They were great. Happy to talk for a minute. I got him to sign it."

There was a large scrawled signature in Sharpie over the bottom of the set list. It was illegible.

"Who? Who signed it?"

"Mike Love."

I thanked Isaac again. I had no doubt about accepting the present. Isaac's intent was clear and I was touched. He had gone on a quest and was literally giving me the gift of love.

We were going to look after each other.

DOING THERAPY WITH SOMEONE who has been sexually abused often raises challenges that lie at the boundary between a therapeutic relationship and a relationship in the real world.

Every three months, I get a magazine in the mail from the College of Physicians and Surgeons. I flip right past the articles about maintaining proper records and when to report a concern about a patient's driving, straight to the Report of the Disciplinary Committee. There I find the summaries of the worst offenses of physicians, the ones who failed to maintain professional boundaries. Sometimes they are colleagues I have known. They did the things you can't do with patients: had sex, accepted loans, exploited or assaulted the people who trusted them with their care. The harm to patients is obvious. For the doctors, it is the ultimate shame.

Relationships that involve categorical asymmetries in power (parent-child, police officer-citizen, teacher-student) always carry the risk of exploitation and abuse. Relationships between health care professionals and their patients carry all of that risk and, by their nature, gaze intently and intimately at one person's most private attributes, without any reciprocal sharing by the other. It is a relationship that requires great trust by patients and great respect and responsibility by providers. The stakes are so high with Isaac, whose trouble starts with sexual assault and exploitation, that a handshake will probably be the only time we touch.

So, what should I do when Isaac offers a gift? When I trained, I was taught to decline gifts as kindly as possible and then to explore what was behind the gesture. It's a sensible approach, but I haven't stuck to it. Too many times, I said no and then spent weeks or longer trying to repair the harm that the hurt did. But yes can screw things up when we accept gifts too. So, I bumble along, trying to make the best choices, always aware that I may be getting it wrong.

At one of our Monday meetings, Jon and I talk about the boundaries that we observe as therapists.

"Do you ever refuse gifts?" I ask.

"Rarely. I've hardly ever been offered anything that had enough monetary value that it felt inappropriate. Once a patient was considering buying me a watch and I said not to. That would feel wrong, even if it was chump change to them. But if someone brings a bottle of wine at Christmas or a cup of coffee, I just say thanks ... Actually, that's not right, I sometimes let a patient know that I have a routine about when I drink coffee or eat, so I appreciate the gesture, but next time don't get me a coffee. Feel free to bring one for yourself though."

"I just say thanks. But when we were trained, they made a big deal about gifts. One teacher said he would accept a coffee but never drink it – the consumption was too laden with symbolic meaning."

"Like letting it sit there going cold isn't." Jon snorted. "You know I have sipped on a coffee I didn't like because a patient didn't know that I like skim milk in it and it didn't feel right to complain about the gift. Mrs. Hunter didn't raise any rude children."

"I've said no to things, and it has really been hurtful," I recalled. "The worst was when a patient invited me to their recital or art show or something like that. It is personal and meaningful, and it can do some harm to decline, although I'm better at declining than I was when I started out."

"Do you always say no?"

"I went to a recital when I was first starting out in practice." I felt like I was confessing. "I realized as soon as I was there that it didn't feel right. It was not part of our relationship; I had wandered out beyond the boundary. A therapy relationship is a special thing, and I didn't realize clearly at that point that it is also a very specific thing. You can't have a therapy relationship and have another kind of relationship too ... Actually, the same patient used to want to talk on the phone. I had long phone conversations in the evening because she was suicidal or just very upset or whatever. I have never done that since, because I realized there needs to be a limit."

"That is something I tell residents. You can't have two kinds of relationship. Your patient can't also be your lawyer, or your business partner, or lover, or even friend."

"That's true. I had another patient who thought we were friends and ended her therapy when I said no, I'm not your friend. I'm your psychiatrist. I try to be friendly, but this is a different kind of relationship. It is not a friendship. Friends are on an equal footing, and we can't be."

"I also say that therapeutic relationships that work aren't all that common and are very valuable. In that way this is better than a friendship," he added. "I had a couple of patients I would speak to for long calls after hours or on the weekend too. I don't do that anymore."

"Is it ever a problem that you don't?"

"Not for me. It is really clear for me now. When a therapeutic relationship crosses a line like that, it becomes less effective. I feel compromised, or beholden, or coerced somehow and that takes away my freedom to do what I need to as a therapist."

"Funny," I said, "the boundaries are supposed to protect the patient. But you're saying you feel coerced in some circumstances ... That happened to me with hugging. I don't hug a lot in real life, so I was very aware that with a couple of patients who want a hug, say at the end of a session, that it felt like I was being pressured to do something I was uncomfortable with. Again, that was back at the beginning. I don't do that anymore, and now it feels pretty easy to decline and explain why if I'm asked. I think back then I didn't want to hurt anyone's feelings."

"Yeah, I felt the same. Another thing I tell the residents is, if you wouldn't feel comfortable telling your supervisor about something, don't do it."

"So those are pretty clear rules. Don't have two relationships. Don't do things that you wouldn't speak freely about."

"Although, as you say that, I realize I'm full of shit. I have patients who are colleagues – doctors who refer patients to me or vice versa, who I also see as patients. So those are two relationships. So far, it seems to have worked out okay. But I don't see everyone who asks, so I guess I am making some choices about what I think will be 'safe' from a boundaries perspective and what won't. I don't really know explicitly what my criteria are though."

We both fall silent for a few seconds.

"I think now that the patient who ended her therapy because I wouldn't say we were friends was very sensitive to the power differential. She needed us to either have a more equal relationship or to say that we did. I didn't address that at the time. So that was a therapy mistake."

"Often I think gifts, hugs, extra calls, and so forth are because a patient wants to know they are special, or that the relationship is special."

"Or gratitude. Sometimes a gift is just a thank you."

Jon spoke more emphatically as he figured out what he thought. "The thing is that you need to know what it means to the patient. It doesn't really matter what your teacher told you thirty years ago. It isn't the rule that matters the most. It is what the patient means by it. If we really believe what we teach about patient-centered care, that should be the first rule: try to figure out what this means to your patient ... I had a patient who gave me things that she had made herself. Creative things. She was a person with terrible self-esteem, who had always felt very unworthy, and so the idea that she could create something that someone else would value was revolutionary for her. That was a positive outcome of therapy. Imagine if she were to give me that and my response was to say, 'I don't accept gifts.' That would be a horrible repetition of the sort of events that made her miserable in the first place."

"So you wouldn't have any qualms about the set list."

"That is a gift of such shared meaning. It would be awful to turn it away. There is no coercion there, nor exploitation."

More silence.

"But psychotherapists do terrible things. A lot of the names in the Discipine Committee report are psychotherapists who have had sex with their patients. We have to be mindful of rationalizing. You know, I *really* like the set list. So that could cloud my judgment."

"Yeah, I suppose. The extreme transgressions seem straightforward to me. Just don't do that stuff. It is the gray zone in the middle where there are never going to be rules that save you. You need to keep the patient in mind. Work at trying to understand what is in their mind. See the lines when you are getting close. Feel comfortable saying, 'No, that's a line I don't cross, but we can talk about it.'"

"Do you think this is just about therapy or do the same things apply in other parts of medicine?"

"For sure it applies elsewhere. And some of the same principles apply. Don't have a business relationship, don't date, all that stuff. But I think the parts that are harder to see are how subtler kinds of exploitation or mistreatment slip into a treatment relationship without thinking about it. What would be an example? Two patients fail to follow through on an important test. One you make a point of calling to see what happened. The other you let slip. I don't think it is random. You are reacting to your relationship with that person. Stuff like that happens more for people with trauma and who have more troubling relationships. A doctor or nurse feels a little relief when they don't come back ... I guess I am off on a tangent. I'm not talking about gifts and boundaries anymore."

"Just a short tangent. Because if you now imagine a gift, the same gift might feel different coming from those two people. It might mean something different to them. So, the same gift might be different coming from them ..."

"Did we figure anything out?"

"The figuring process is ongoing. That is always the conclusion. You can't figure this stuff out once and for all. You need to keep paying attention."

13

"It ends here"

Sixteen years into our long conversation, Isaac's mother died. She had been weak and getting sicker for years and spent her last four weeks in a palliative care hospice. He spent a few days afterward in her condo in the Bronx, a few blocks from where he grew up. It was crammed with expensive curios that were of no interest to him, little paintings, fancy rugs, and seemingly thousands of books. He was trying to sort the things that might have some sentimental value to her grandchildren from the things that were expensive but meaningless junk.

The sorting was too much for one person but no one else volunteered. Isaac's younger brother, Scott, lived too far away. His older brother, Neil, had refused to have anything to do with their mother for decades. When describing her, Isaac occasionally called his mother "the insect," an unpleasant nickname that conveyed the lack of warmth he felt both from her and for her. I had learned over time that the inhuman identifier also signaled a troubled and complicated emotional connection. What Neil called her is unprintable.

Over the years, I heard about Isaac's mother in two ways. In stories of his youth, her role usually consisted of her absence, the times when she wasn't present, didn't notice, didn't respond, or didn't think to protect Isaac or his brothers. More recent stories were different. His father has been dead for decades. Isaac regularly traveled back to the Bronx to take care of his mother's finances. He made sure that there were investments to cover her retirement needs and her expensive tastes. He explained and re-explained why she needed to sign a document or make a choice for her bank or her broker. Isaac spoke to his mother on the phone most weeks, always him calling her. He found the calls almost unbearable. She was self-involved, opinionated, seeking pity or sympathy, complaining. Isaac talked back; he didn't mind being rude and it seemed to make no difference. Sometimes he held the phone at arm's length while she spoke. He was passive-aggressive and plain-old-aggressive, but he called.

When Isaac's mother was admitted to the hospice at the end of her illness, Isaac stayed with her most of the time, alone in an uncomfortable armchair by her bed. Her physical suffering touched a nerve, and he advocated for pain relief in his usual fierce style.

"My mother is suffering. Look at her. The medication is not working," he said to the young doctor who was visiting the hospice to make rounds. It was the first time they had met and Isaac started the conversation in a manner that was calm but direct.

"I will see what we have her on. We can probably adjust the dose."

"What do you mean *probably*? Just crank up the dose until she isn't hurting."

Isaac moved from calm to insistent. The young doctor responded to the hostility he perceived with as much balance as he could muster. "These are powerful drugs that can also do harm. I'll try to find the right balance."

"There's no balance to find. Just take away her pain. It doesn't matter if it kills her."

"We ... we don't kill people, but we're here to help your mother feel comfortable."

Isaac looked across the room at the other patient, asleep now but oblivious even when she was awake. He glanced up at the security camera in the hall that could be seen through the doorway. It took one step to be precisely in the young doctor's face, and one quick move to grab his lapels and push his back to the wall.

"I don't think you understand your job, and I don't think you under-stand your problem. This woman needs relief."

She died within a couple of days. Isaac bluffed and threatened his way through the repercussions of assaulting and threatening the doctor who was trying to care for his dying mother. Nothing came of it. And then he was left to sort through her overstuffed apartment.

"You were there for your mother in a way that she was not there for you."

"Don't get the idea that it was warm. I couldn't stand her. She was so self-involved right to the end."

"But you were still there. It makes me think of how you protect your children. Of course, you *are* warm for them ... I just mean that somehow you have determined that the people who rely on you are going to get bet-ter treatment than you got. As if you are saying 'it ends here.'"

Isaac looked unconvinced.

I leaned forward to emphasize my point. "I think you had determined that 'it ends here' before you met me. Your experience as a parent says so. But I also think that is an example of what we are aiming for. Even if we can't fix your brain or relieve your pain the way that I wish we could, we can at least acknowledge that it is an achievement not to pass it on to someone else."

It would have been easier for Isaac to abandon "the insect" as Neil had done, but he didn't. He would never admit to love or even to loyalty, but he took care of his mother. His motivation may have been as simple as a rule: you look after your family. Kids often choose paths that are defined by their parents' actions – either replicating what they have learned or adamantly choosing the opposite. Maybe it was the latter, an imperative to care for and protect family without conditions or reward, the opposite of his experience.

I don't know Isaac's mother's story. It has felt beside the point of our conversation. But I know she has one, and that knowing it would help make sense of what it was like for her in that family in the Bronx in the 1950s and '60s. Her story would not relieve her responsibility or excuse her absences, any more than Isaac's experience of her makes her culpable – the goal of understanding is not to differentiate the victims and the villains; it is to understand.

There was nothing nice or warm about Isaac's care for his mother. Sometimes that is the best that a person who has been harmed and unprotected can do, to choose the opposite path – to be there for her rather than not to be there at all. That is one way to make sure that a cycle of trauma ends.

TRAUMA'S HARM PASSES DOWN generations. The clearest evidence of this is from crimes against humanity, whose harm reverberates to the second and third generation. Children and grandchildren of the victims of these crimes experience depression, addiction, death by suicide, and other harms much more often than those whose ancestors escaped that fate. This damage is observed in the descendants of Indigneous children separated from their families and culture, dehumanized, and brutalized in Canadian Indian residential schools; in the children and grandchildren of victims of the Holocaust; and in the offspring of former Japanese sexual slaves in World War II ("comfort women"). The traumas of individual families, the result of individual harm and invalidation rather than malignant cultural forces, also passes down generations.

Harm is sometimes transmitted in obvious ways, by parents who are too depressed or intoxicated to engage in the difficult job of parenting, or who are too frightened or angry to keep a child's mind in their own mind. My grandmother, Edie, told me about growing up on the Canadian Prairie with her father, a stretcher bearer in the Boer War before they emigrated from England to Canada, who then joined the No. 3 Canadian Field Ambulance in World War I. He came back afraid of lightning storms, hiding under the bed, throwing things, and spending "some time at the Psychopathic." Edie's mother was pretty tough, and kind enough, and did the job of parenting on her own, I guess. Edie married Max, who had some charisma and a job where he got to wear a hat and tie, but Max tended to drink his paychecks, leaving Edie and my young dad to scramble to find coal to burn to heat their rented apartment (or hotel room for a while, when they lost the apartment) in Winnipeg during the winter. Enter the next generation: Max stopped drinking when my mother told him that he wouldn't be allowed to visit his grandchildren if he continued. Sometimes, someone is able to decide "it ends here."

Harm is also transmitted in ways that are less obvious. Dr. Amy Bombay of the School of Nursing at Dalhousie University has a PhD in psychology and neuroscience and is Ojibway from Rainy River First Nations. Among her several studies exploring the intergenerational effects of the Indian residential school system in Canada, one describes a cycle in which the offspring of survivors of those schools respond to past discrimination by finding their Indigenous heritage to be central to their identity and, in turn, tend to attribute others' hostility to discrimination and to see it as a threat to their well-being, which feeds into higher levels of depressive symptoms. I can hear Isaac's experiences echoing in this dynamic cycle. One thing leads to another. When he is accused of overreacting to what he perceives as harmful intent, he argues back that his eyes are open whereas others are blind or in denial.

Sometimes, the effects of trauma literally get under the skin. Adult children of Holocaust survivors have not only experienced more childhood trauma than their peers (mostly the emotional abuse and neglect that results from their parents' post-traumatic stress disorder, as happened to Marlene), but also have more stress hormones circulating in their systems, contributing to chronic diseases of wear and tear, like heart disease and stroke. In both the survivors of the Holocaust and their children, regulation of genes (by molecules that determine which genes are turned on and which turned off) is altered, evidence that traumatic experiences that occur before conception may possibly affect genetically controlled biological processes that influence disease.

Trauma itself may pass from one generation to the next. To understand how that works, first burn this non sequitur into your consciousness: let's say one out of every five hundred medical students becomes a pediatric radiologist, reading X-rays in a children's hospital. On the other hand, every single pediatric radiologist has gone to medical school. Going to medical school vastly increases the likelihood that you will become a pediatric radiologist, but that career is still a very uncommon outcome of medical school.

The evidence that perpetrators of trauma have been traumatized as children is similar. Among perpetrators of child sexual abuse, the likelihood they themselves experienced sexual abuse as a child is high, and yet by far most victims of childhood sexual abuse do not go on to abuse others. Most often, it ends with the victim. I emphasize that because Isaac has suffered greatly by keeping his abuse a secret, in part because he expects that if others knew, then they would become afraid of him. His experience of himself, repeated over and over to me, is that "I am fucked up beyond repair." Although he has never posed a danger to a child, in fact quite the opposite, it is a small step from seeing oneself as fucked up to expecting others to see one as fucked up *and dangerous*. The fear and the stigma are powerful.

Much more commonly, the consequences of childhood adversity interfere with parenting in subtler ways. Depressive symptoms or intoxication make a father less available in moments that matter. An innocent interaction that triggers a memory of trauma leads a mother to react to what is going on in her head instead of what is happening in front of her, "spacing out" in a way that temporarily disconnects her from her child. People miss out on validating experiences growing up that would have made it second nature to provide a validating environment for their kids, so their efforts are clumsy and inconsistent.

I believe that harm can diminish over generations rather than perpetually repeat. It *can* end. One bit of solace that I have found over decades of doing therapy with people like Isaac is that even though personal healing is hard to come by, my patients are often better parents than their parents were. They make choices that serve their own kids well.

The "victims and villains" narrative doesn't help. Sometimes I invoke that narrative as a corrective for patients who are so embroiled in guilt, shame, and self-blame that they can't appreciate that someone else who had much more power harmed them at a time when they were in no position to stop it. "It wasn't your fault. You were a kid. He harmed you. You couldn't stop it." Even then, it is better to focus on what the other person did than to call him evil. The "victims and villains" story is usually inaccurate or at least incomplete. The story of what the insect did omits what happened to the insect. It is the truth, but it isn't the whole truth. Beyond that, it silences the other side of Isaac's ambivalence. Because it would appear that, in spite of what he says, Isaac felt something like love for his mother. Understanding Isaac requires seeing that love, in addition to the harm he suffered while she was somewhere else.

Solutions call for understanding rather than blame. The world does not comprise good parents versus bad ones or damaged and sick people versus normal ones. When Isaac holds the receiver at arm's length from his ear while his mother talks, is he arrogant and hostile or doing the best he can to support a woman he finds intolerable? When he assaults the doctor at the hospice, is he an advocate or a menace? Are his eyes open to threats and indifference from health care providers, or does he only see what he already expects? It's always two things. There are days when I can't do much better than to choose an answer. On a good day, Isaac and I find a way to live with the tension between opposites.

14
"Help me"

Scotty, Isaac, and Neil were sitting around the table eating their breakfast cereal. Isaac was ten.

"What's this?" asked their mother, holding up the message pad from beside the telephone and shaking it. The message on the pad could not be clearer or more mysterious. "HELP ME" in block letters was obviously written by a child, but the boys' mother couldn't tell which one.

No one answered. The expressions on their faces didn't give anything away.

"Right then." Their mother ripped the top page off the pad and threw the crumpled ball into the garbage. As far as Isaac knows, that is as far as her curiosity extended. It was as close as he came to asking a grown-up to help him get away from the young man next door.

"Two years later, there was the thing with my bicycle ..."

He had told me that story before. He was alone in the garage of their house for a long time and when he came out, the garage looked like a crime scene. No one had been hurt, but he had smashed his bicycle almost beyond recognition. He had thrown it against the floor and hit it with a cinder block and with a hammer. He had separated its parts and bent its spokes and rims, ripped open the fake-leather seat, smashed reflectors and a mirror into shards. Isaac had never seen his father as angry as he was when he came home that night and saw the bicycle's remains

"No one ever asked, 'What's going on? Why did you do that?' It was just bad behavior. I was punished and then my brothers had bikes and I didn't. I never had a bike again."

"Were you hoping someone would ask?"

"Obviously."

My brow scrunched up in protest. "I'm not sure it was obvious. But clearly something was wrong. You hadn't done anything like that before ..."

"It was a clear fucking communication."

"It was a dramatic, angry communication. It was also your own bike. You were the only one that got hurt."

"It was clear."

We got onto the subject of asking for help because two weeks earlier, Isaac asked if I would help him to kill himself, although he knows the answer. Usually he avoids the question, because forcing me to refuse, again, to prescribe a drug that will end his life sucks all of the oxygen out of our conversation. Neither of us wants that.

But on that day, he was tired and sore and didn't see how things were going to change except to get harder. He was clear that he wasn't planning suicide just then, but he wanted to know if I would help when the time came, sooner than I think.

My answer wasn't very good. "I think the idea that I would help you is important. It is not hard to find a way to die; it is not like I am withholding the only means you would have. So, I'm guessing that it is not really the prescription we are talking about; it's more like some ultimate test of whether I'll help you when you need it."

"It's not as easy as you think. And why should I die in some horrible way when you could give me a good death?"

If this was an ultimate test of helping, I was failing. Yet another unanswered plea for help.

Isaac and I can trace a path from his anonymous, almost silent, plea (the message pad), to a dramatic but ambiguous and hostile request for curiosity and help (the bike), to a demand that is both clear and certain to be refused (the poison). And then, three years later, there was the email – clear, heartfelt, and possible: "I've always asked you for everything you have, no half measures, and once again, I need you to help me understand the damage that I am."

It is deeply dissatisfying that Isaac and I have not yet succeeded in our effort to allow him to heal, but I take solace in knowing that some things change. Directly asking for help can be overwhelmingly difficult because of what it risks: the harm that can come from revealing a vulnerability or from another person's rejection or indifference.

I am doing everything I can to respond. We're not done yet, but we're getting there.

HEALTH HAPPENS BETWEEN PEOPLE. Illness and disease emerge from interactions that are harmful or protective, that model and encourage self-care or the opposite. One person fails to wash his hands; another gets sick. Governments that devise and enforce health policy and corporations whose products harm or protect consumers are composed of people, informed by people, directed by people – one through their votes, another through their profits. Even diseases of dumb bad luck, like many cancers, are detected or not, treated or not, cured or not, because of the choices and efforts of people, often by people who are not the ones with the tumor. As much as our current reflex is to think that disease is fundamentally biological, it makes as much sense to say both disease and illness are fundamentally social.

Unless the patient is unconscious, health care always takes place within relationships – it is transactional. With only a few exceptions, the transactions between people that comprise health care begin with one kind: one person asks for help and another person responds. Simple. But what if the most significant events in a person's early life, events that shape his health and health care, have themselves undermined his ability to ask for help?

More is known about how kids speak about sexual abuse – or don't – than about other forms of adversity. Most children keep it to themselves, or if they tell anyone, they tell a peer rather than an adult. Unsurprisingly, but unfortunately, the more severe the experience of sexual abuse, the less likely a child will speak to an adult. Isaac's experience of not speaking of what happened until he was grown is the norm. Other patients have told me about speaking up only to have a parent tell them they are lying or ask them what they did to encourage it. It doesn't have to be that way. Kids are more likely to speak up to adults who are supportive and who are curious about their well-being. Adolescents who are referred to social agencies say that whether or not they share their experiences depends mostly on trust and feeling that they are in a safe place. We could be better listeners. But secrecy is the norm.

It isn't just kids. As adults, men who were sexually abused as boys silence themselves or feel silenced. They have many reasons: mistrust of those who would know, a sense that their masculinity is at risk, the intense emotions, and difficulty naming the experience as abuse. Isaac is not alone in waiting decades. Women are similarly reluctant to speak about sexual violence, expecting, for good reason, to be blamed or not to be believed. Asking for help may be an even greater hurdle. Support resources are limited. One cannot be guaranteed a sensitive response. There are even more barriers for people of color who experience discrimination and for immigrants who face social isolation, language barriers, and fears of deportation. Ongoing family violence complicates the consequences of past experiences for many women and makes it even harder to speak.

As a boy, Isaac needed and wanted help. In a sense, one of the major themes of his therapy has been learning to voice a need for help. He was initially too frightened and ashamed to reveal what had happened; he went to great lengths to avoid being discovered. On the other hand, he wrote HELP ME on a pad. It was the best he could do, but without a curious, concerned response, the request was doomed.

Asking for what one needs assertively and effectively is a difficult skill. It is hard to pick your moments, to feel entitled to what you are requesting, and to avoid sounding aggressive. Many of us get through life without ever getting very good at it. It is not surprising that when one learns at an early age that asking for help with overwhelming threats and injuries is impossible, it undermines the development of assertive help seeking for other needs as well. Usually, early adversity influences help seeking by either squashing it, as it has for Isaac, or by amplifying it – some former victims of abuse are virtually constantly seeking help of one kind or another.

Isaac is fiercely independent. He doesn't ask for much. He doesn't reveal much about his need when he does ask. In a health care setting, he either asks for nothing (by not going there in the first place) or is likely to make a demand and to feel that his need is self-evident. If the professional doesn't understand or disagrees, it sets up a conflict that may be infused with more hostility and defensiveness than is necessary, as happened with the young doctor at his mother's hospice. His request for my help is an extraordinary exception. In a sense it is a gift he makes to me, to entrust me with responding to the parts of him that it is not safe to reveal elsewhere.

For others, it sometimes goes the other way, with demands for help and attention that are enough to overwhelm almost anybody.

Jon told me about a patient he was once asked to see in the Emergency Department.

"They called me because she was 'agitated.' No more info than that, but a clear sense of urgency. I was expecting someone confused by delirium, maybe, but nope. Gloria was tearing strips off everyone in her path. The ED staff had no bandwidth left, because she was yelling complaints about everybody and everything: The nurse 'blew it' when he drew blood; the X-ray tech was asking her to lie in an impossible position; the admitting clerk misspelled her name; and the residents sure as shit weren't the staff doctors that she deserved. So that was essentially the consult: 'Jon, you gotta get her outta here!'"

"Turns out Gloria had come to the ED because she had been waking up with drenching night sweats. She had a big lymph node in her neck and the imaging looked like Hodgkin's lymphoma."

"So cancer, but curable," I interjected.

"The plan was to admit her to the hospital to confirm the diagnosis and test to see if it had spread. It took a while to even get a word in sideways, after I introduced myself. She was furious that psychiatry had been called. 'I'm not crazy! I'll tell you who's crazy ... whoever called you guys!' I sent the resident away because 'sending in the minions' (Gloria's words) just made everything worse. She was not going to stand for the implication that she was not worth the 'real doctor's' time.

"Once she was admitted, she got fewer visits from psychiatry than she would have otherwise because my time is tighter than the residents and also because it became clear there was no point showing up unless I had a lot of time to spend with her, and I don't often have a full hour free. But I went when I could and stayed in touch with the nurses and docs by dropping into the nursing station for a few minutes, even if I didn't go see Gloria herself. When I had time, I sat down by the bedside and let Gloria wind down without interrupting her – no refutations, no argument, and precious little clarification, even when her rant became hard to follow, as it often did because Gloria needed to be heard but wasn't thinking about how I was going to understand her. After she had spoken her piece, each time I told her that I believed being in hospital was not good for her because, although she had so much pain and worry, she was also too angry and upset to feel cared for there. Rarely, I had enough of an opening to suggest that she was probably scared by the disease, but that the hospital, with all its rules and a constant stream of new faces, was scaring her even more. The medical team agreed it was safe and was only too happy to look after her as an outpatient as soon as she agreed to go home.

"Her time in the chemo clinic wasn't much better, but she was only there for a few hours every third week, so she and the staff tolerated each other more easily. The nurses figured her out and made adjustments. For example, they altered usual clinic processes to reduce the amount of time Gloria spent waiting, to reduce her frustration and avoid altercations. Gloria, for her part, over time came to appreciate these accommodations, and started to arrive early to make things easier for the nurses, seeing as they were taking a few extra steps for her sake. I saw her in the clinic while she was getting chemo, 'just droppin' in to see how you're doin',' and smoothed out conflicts when they arose, often just by letting the nurses vent. The chemo worked and Gloria went ten years without a recurrence. In spite of these 'wins,' Gloria never felt that her oncologist was on her side; she figured that she irritated him (which was right) and that he avoided her when he could (also right). When he told her she was 'cured' and didn't need any more treatment or monitoring, she felt rejected.

"There was no position on the cancer ward or in the chemo clinic that felt safe or comfortable to Gloria. She resented the doctors' power to control the treatments she needed. She tried to seize power but in the process alienated the people who wanted to help her.

"Eventually I learned what that was about. It was heartrending, once I got to know her, because it seemed like she was reliving the situation she grew up in. She was raised on a big farm and her parents treated the kids like cheap labor. She was often lonely in spite of all the people around and the neglect was severe ... interrupted only by her father's physical abuse and yelling. If he was paying attention, he was frightening. Her 'agitation' was an imitation of his way of being in control. So, when she was scared and sick, Gloria drove people away instead of inviting their help. She was in desperate need of connection and almost impossible to approach ... but she got rid of her cancer, so that's something. It took a lot of tolerance and effort on both sides, but she did get the treatment and it worked."

Effective health care emerges from collaboration between patients and providers. It is relational. There are many impediments to achieving full collaboration – most are systemic and cultural barriers that are imposed by health care's formal and informal organizations. Trauma just makes it worse.

15
Under siege

Isaac lives like a wounded soldier under siege. He is vigilant for what hides behind the next corner, whether in his mind or in the world. Unlike people who have the luxury of waiting to see what life will bring, Isaac always expects that he will need to fight and fears that his body will be too sore and exhausted to protect him. Constantly evaluating his inner and outer worlds for threats and resources while navigating a painful chronic disease leads to mixed-up sequences of experiences. We never get to deal with one thing at a time.

Isaac has been invited to join the negotiating team in a major labor dispute. It is a long-term project. I don't understand the details, but he is passionate about the challenge and cares about the issues. The prospect of being able to play to his strengths is good for him, so it is discouraging when he concludes that he can't do it. The gut pain from Crohn's disease and the much more severe pain in his right knee from arthritis is too much to allow him to tolerate the demanding schedule that would be required. Setting aside the offer, Isaac returns to his plan to eventually die by suicide. Not yet, but when he can no longer tolerate the pain.

Vivid memories of childhood abuse intrude into Isaac's thoughts. If nothing else was going on, we would probably be talking about his job, but he can't follow any thread for long without it being interrupted by a spasm of pain or intrusive memories that he usually doesn't want to describe. We talk about the only two things that have helped over the years: drugs and therapy. Both are anesthetic, drugs in the obvious way, our relationship more mysteriously.

One day, Isaac walks in using a cane, a first. The knee pain is too preoccupying to talk about anything else. It is an awful conversation because he has nothing to say except how much it hurts.

"I'm not going to make it."

I have virtually nothing to say at all; the best I can do is to try to look receptive to whatever he wants to share. So, I am relieved that the next couple of times we meet, Isaac tells me that he has had dreams. That almost always opens a window of some sort.

The voice of the young man next door calls Isaac from the basement.

Isaac wakes in a sweat and goes downstairs to have a cigarette, watching the windows as if it is inevitable that an intruder will appear.

The next time we meet he has had a dream in which a different voice says, "There is no one calling you." There is no other image or plot.

"Was it my voice, or someone else you recognize?"

"No. I don't recognize the voice."

"But it was an intervention. It was meant to counteract the other dream."

"I guess."

"You are the dreamer. You made the dream. You intervened to reassure yourself about the other dream."

"I don't think so. I don't control my dreams."

"Sure. Dreams don't seem under our control. My point is that the expression comes from you. Some part of yourself is not just reliving old terrors. It is intervening to help you."

He misses the next two scheduled appointments because of repeated migraines and pain in his gut and knee. I wonder if I was pushing too hard, and it made things worse. If our relationship can relieve pain when it is working well, it can also aggravate it when it isn't.

There are signs of a growing bowel obstruction. Isaac tried to reach his gastroenterologist, who is out of town at a conference. The doctor sent an email suggesting that Isaac call the surgeon he knows from previous encounters or go to the Emergency Department. Isaac was enraged by that response – someone should be there for him. He tries to cool down, wanting to avoid severing the connection he values with his gastroenterologist out of anger.

When I see Isaac again, he uses our time to plan the conversation with his gastroenterologist, working out how to let him know what he thinks is wrong with the doctor's coverage plan without antagonizing him. It seems to work. He sees the gastroenterologist, speaks his piece, and they construct a new plan to increase the dose of his medication. Isaac wants to avoid surgery.

One step forward.

The next week he tells me he thinks he may be up to joining the labor negotiating team after all. And then he reports two new dreams.

A small male face with a brush cut gets larger and larger. It is the predator next door.

A wild young boy who looks "like he was raised by wolves" has blue skin.

"I know what that was about. When I was six, Neil and I missed school for a year because we had ringworm all over. They painted our skin with this blue stuff."

"Gentian violet. It is a treatment for fungal infections."

"Yeah, exactly. And our hair was shaved. We looked like freaks. We ran wild with no supervision. We did whatever we wanted. It was crazy. That was first grade so I didn't learn to read well. I was still a freak when we went back to school. I was older than all of the other kids in the new class but I couldn't read. And we got the ringworm from a fucking cat our father forced on us. I didn't want it but he was trying to force me to get over a fear of cats."

Isaac practically spat the last words out. After the two dreams, he had a continuous migraine for ten days and missed his appointments. However, within a month, the increased dose of medication seemed to be working. The gut and knee pain was subsiding. Isaac had made some calls and joined the negotiating team.

And so it goes, one step forward, one step back, sometimes more. Threats from the past are briefly interrupted by intervention and hope. Isaac puts extraordinary effort into overcoming the reflex of rage he experiences when he feels abandoned. This effort is new. But when he dares to experience relief or plan for the future, pain and terrible memories intrude once again as if to say, "Not so fast, boy, we're not done with you yet."

"I WAS TALKING TO my brother Neil. He was reminding me of the things we did in our neighborhood when we were just young, ten or eleven. All this dangerous stuff: grabbing onto the bumper of a bus when the streets were icy in the winter and sliding behind it, sometimes going down to a rail-yard where you could hitch a ride on the trains when they slowed down.

"Then he was talking about some things that I don't remember, and I realized that I have almost no memory of fourth grade. I can't remember who my teacher was or who was in my class. Nothing."

The next time we met, Isaac was waiting in a chair in the hallway outside my office. The hallway is not wide; it requires respecting others' space. A patient of one of the other psychiatrists was pacing erratically. He was young and he looked like he hadn't showered in a few days. His clothes were a mess. His eyes darted back and forth. He looked a little unhinged.

I gestured to Isaac that I was ready for him to come in.

"I could take him if I had to," he said menacingly as he came into my office and sat down.

Isaac was carrying a leather bag by its handles and set it on the floor. As he reached inside the bag, he asked "Do you wonder what I'm going to pull out of here?" The question was vague, but seemed intended to raise a little fear.

He paused and then brought out a picture of Neil and him from when he was four or five years old. He wanted me to know Neil.

"He protected me. There was this time when we were both in trouble at school. I can't remember what we did. Neil said, 'Just be quiet and let me do the talking. I won't let them strap you.'"

Isaac leaned back into his chair and took a minute to choose his words.

"I'm ready to go back to what we talked about before. There was a blindfold ..."

He picked up the story of a terrible event that had occurred in the basement of the young man's house next door, just where he had left off several weeks earlier, as if there was no interruption. He told the whole story this time while I just listened.

"So it happened, but it doesn't feel like it happened to me. It was some other kid."

Over the next couple of weeks Isaac went back to the story to repeat parts or fill in details. We talked about how difficult it was to speak about these events and the circumstances that allowed him to do that. It was important that I found him a bit dangerous, he needed to be formidable. It was also important to invoke the presence of Neil. Isaac needed a protector.

Then we talked about his "in-between" connection to traumatic memories, as if the victim of the harm was a person who was sort of him and sort of someone else. I kept going back to that tension, thinking that coming to realize that the memories are truly his own would be a step toward healing, although a painful one.

"I had that dream again, with the bats swooping around this room. Maybe it was a cell. But you were with me in the room, on the other side of the bats. They were between us."

In the dream, I am an adult and Isaac is a child. I point to the creatures and name them and explain to him about them. When we come together to talk this way, the creatures are afraid and fly out of an opening in the back of the cell. It was such a good new ending to the dream, I must have smiled.

The next session there was another variation on the dream.

"This time there are three people in the cell: me, my father, and you. I'm a child. There are no bats. You are explaining to my father that even though he cannot see the creatures, they are there."

I felt buoyed by the optimism of the previous version of the dream and the creativity of this one. It seemed like Isaac was playing with the possibilities of the dream; that the bats could be present or absent, visible or invisible, that he could have a protector and a teacher. So I took a chance.

"If you could go into that dream as an adult, if you were there in that cell as an adult, with Isaac the boy ... If you had a chance to say something or do something for that boy ... What would you do?"

It was a setup. I was hoping, too obviously I suppose, that he would want to protect or comfort the boy.

"I'd exterminate him."

"I'D EXTERMINATE HIM" took my breath away. I had been inspired by the sense that Isaac and I had found a moment in our relationship that was secure enough that we could play. I had dared to hope that we were briefly of one mind, but those words punctured my optimism. In retrospect, I recognize that I had set him up; my question was a manipulation. I was like a parent playing-acting with their kid who wrecks a perfect moment by trying to make sure that the fable ends with a moral. My "moral" was about adopting an adult, comforting, protective stance toward the scared and hurting kid Isaac once was. I had lost sight of what Isaac wanted, which was relief for that kid. I let my wishes get in the way of listening well and responding to his cues. Given the option, he would put that boy out of his misery.

By now I hope it is obvious that this is not a heroic story of overcoming odds or even a reassuring story of healing; I am doing my best to convey something close to the truth about a complicated man and my relationship with him. It doesn't always go well.

PSYCHOTHERAPY IS NOT ALWAYS so complicated and inefficient. These days, people who need therapy and are able to find a therapist (which is no small feat) usually find one who is skilled in a time-limited therapy that has a name and an abbreviation: cognitive-behavioral therapy (CBT), interpersonal psychotherapy (IPT), dialectical-behavior therapy (DBT), and others. These forms of therapy are described in manuals so that they can be taught and learned with some consistency. Therapists have specific skills and, ideally, stick to the principles of their model, which differ from one type of therapy to the next. For example, CBT starts with the premise that how you think affects how you feel; IPT starts with the premise that loss, conflict, and disconnection in key relationships can cause depression. It would be typical for the therapist and client to meet once a week for about four months. DBT is more intensive and lasts longer because it aims to treat borderline personality disorder, which is a much more challenging and seemingly more permanent problem than most forms of depression. These types of therapy have become the norm because there is good evidence that they work, which comes from randomized controlled trials, the same research design that is used to test drug treatments. Isaac and I are doing something different. It doesn't have a name or a manual. One psychotherapy expert, Jon Allen, playfully calls it plain old therapy (POT). Plain old therapy is good for problems that don't fall in neat diagnostic bins, especially when building trust and a working relationship is a big job from the start. It is a form of therapy that helps each of us to learn to keep the other in mind. However, it is harder to know if you are making the right therapeutic choices when you do plain old therapy.

At one of our Monday meetings, Jon and I are talking about times that psychotherapy has felt hopeless.

Jon starts. "One patient comes to mind because this is recent. A few years ago, I saw a woman who had a cancer removed. It was a cancer type with a really poor prognosis, but they told her they 'got it all' in surgery. So, she had been told it was a bad cancer, but she had also been told she was disease free, so she began to feel like she was cured. In the meantime, no shit, her husband got ALS, Lou Gehrig's disease, which of course is progressive and incurable and was fairly advanced. So she is his care provider. That was her role, in her mind – the one who is well and looking after him. Now her cancer has come back and they are both officially terminal. They have, I don't know, maybe a year or less. And that crushed her sense of who she was, of what the point was …

"So, I'm seeing her for therapy because she is pretty depressed and completely pessimistic. There's no daylight. And I'm thinking, *Am I doing the right thing here? How is this going to help? She is not wrong to expect the worst.*"

Health care providers usually want to fix things. It's probably why we go into this kind of work. The sometimes enormous limitations on our ability to do that can lead us to feel hopeless. No matter how many times we face the challenge of illness that defies cure, it remains difficult to see that we can be much more useful by relaxing that demand on ourselves: we can lead with empathy instead of problem-solving.

"And then, I think of the stages of coping," Jon continues, "and I say, well, we're not going to fix the cancer or the ALS here, but we can maybe change how you are feeling about it and what you make of this. You might be living differently if you weren't so depressed. Maybe we could try an antidepressant drug – there's enough time for it to work. And maybe we can talk about what you think your role is, what your purpose is right now … Because they have kids who are barely adults who are about to be orphaned, and that matters to her … and that conversation kind of turned things around, because she gets that she is dying but she doesn't want to feel *like this*. So, the situation is hopeless, but then it felt more hopeful. There was some point to trying to do something – helping her kids, and leaving a bit of a legacy. She could work with me, and she could resist withdrawing from others. I guess the cliché is that it is one thing to be dying but it feels worse to be dying alone."

There was a little pause before I spoke. "The last thing you said reminds me of a couple of people, whom I saw for a long time. They have both died since. They both come to mind because they were kind of similar, in that the therapy didn't seem to me to lead to any progress, but they really valued it, so I had to justify to myself why we were doing it. One was really underweight from anorexia nervosa and had lots of medical complications from that ... even had a brain bleed – anyway, she comes to mind because of the thing you said about not dying alone.

"She wasn't dying at the time, but every week was the same thing. She was full of resentment at how others treated her. Every week was a bad week. It was really hard to engage with her. I dreaded the appointments. It seemed like my role was just to be a witness to how badly the world treated her. I tried different ways to turn that into something more constructive but I couldn't turn the trick.

"Yet, she really valued the time. She never missed an appointment and she told me how important it was. And then at some point I said 'You remind me of Sisyphus.' And I told her the story of Sisyphus, who is condemned to push his stone up to the top of the hill; when he gets to the top, the stone rolls back down and he has to push it up again. And he repeats that forever. There is no progress. That is his perpetual punishment for having offended the gods. I can't remember which god. And I said, 'I guess if you have to perpetually push that stone up the hill, it is better not to have to do it alone.' She liked that, and it helped me too."

"Why did you think of Sisyphus?" Jon asked.

"Albert Camus. That was his metaphor for life. He said that is what we are all doing, pushing that rock up the same hill over and over, and our task is to find some meaning or purpose. That purpose is not given, we have to find it or make it." I felt a blush of self-consciousness and averted my eyes. "That is probably not exactly what he said, but it is what I took from it."

There was another pause before Jon spoke. "Remember when you played rugby on the Meds team?"

"Yeah."

"If you got the ball from a scrum and the other team was starting to pile on, you never let it go."

"I never got away either," I acknowledged. "I wasn't any good at running to advance the ball, and I usually didn't think to pass it."

"And you couldn't kick worth shit," Jon added helpfully.

"I just held on. I wasn't very good, but I was tenacious."

"I had an approach to treating patients like that when I first graduated from residency. I was absolutely sure being a good doctor meant taking on the tough cases, persevering, no matter how hard. If I wasn't building an alliance, if they weren't getting better, it was just evidence that I wasn't trying hard enough. That's the message that I took away from my senior supervisors. It didn't feel wrong or risky. It felt like serious business, and I was proud to help out when others wouldn't."

"I see the rugby connection," I said. "It would have been better if I was not so tenacious sometimes."

Jon continued. "It *felt* like I was doing the special good work, but, here's the thing – it didn't always translate into good therapy. I had a patient, Angie, who was very distrustful of the whole idea of therapy. She had tried it before and just felt misunderstood and criticized. But she was so profoundly at odds with the world, always feeling wronged and picking fights, maybe like your anorexic lady, that she was going to try therapy again. It was miserable work. She rejected what I said, insisted that I didn't care or couldn't be trusted. I was constantly trying to prove that I was trustworthy, that I was going to be the exception to her expectations. Each session I would feel like we were building a better alliance – and then I'd get a voicemail message, even before the end of the day, telling me how terrible I was. Next session we'd start again with distrust and me trying to prove my bone fides. Nothing was changing in therapy or in the rest of her life as far as I could tell.

"I became preoccupied with the sessions, sleeping poorly the night before as I anticipated the attack and resenting how my thoughts about the therapy intruded later that day and the next day, and still getting nowhere ... I'm embarrassed to tell you that this went on for years. It was just a 'groundhog day' of her preemptive anger, the best defense is a strong offense, and then retreat until the next time.

"It never helped her. I'm sure the frustration made her worse, and it was definitely bad for me. I needed help, a colleague or supervisor to look at it from the outside. I tried to get another opinion, but Angie distrusted anyone else even more and refused, and I went along with her.

I didn't know how to end the therapy without proving her right, that I was as bad as everyone else who rejected her. It did stop eventually, but it didn't end well.

"More than ten years later I got a kind of cryptic message from Angie, with very little explanation. I guess she was letting me know she was alive, that she had persevered. Or maybe it was a 'Fuck you, I'm doing fine without you.' I don't know. But I know I blew it."

I waited a second before trading stories. "I think about my mistakes too. You learn from mistakes. I keep a woman in my mind who came to get her depression treated once. While I was trying to understand what was going on, it came out that she was sexually abused as a girl and had never spoken about it to anyone. It had been her preference not to speak of it – a stiff upper lip and 'keep your dirty laundry to yourself' sort of attitude. I gave her an alternative, a relationship in which she could speak about things that otherwise were completely buried. It opened Pandora's Box. Intrusive memories and nightmares and panic attacks. It was crippling, and although I worked really hard to treat it and so did she, it didn't get better."

"Post-traumatic stress disorder. You don't think that was there before?" Jon asked.

"She said no and I believe her. So that was a mistake that did a lot of harm."

"Maybe. But you don't know what the alternative would have been. Maybe she would have just quietly killed herself after a few more years. That happens."

I was not convinced. "Maybe. But there is a lot of room for rationalization ... justifying mistakes. I prefer to take it as a cautionary story. Don't open the box unless you are pretty sure you have something better to offer."

"Doctors who never ask about childhood adversity fear the Pandora's Box thing," said Jon. "That's what they expect will happen."

"Usually it doesn't," I replied. "Most people don't blurt much more than they are ready to reveal. Their defenses kick into place. But you can't say never ... I think the thing here was not so much the asking as it was digging deeper after asking. I think it is a cautionary story about the power of psychotherapy. All effective treatments for anything – drugs, surgery, whatever – also have the potential to harm. Therapy is no different. It is an argument against naive psychotherapy."

Psychotherapy is mostly provided in specific modalities of therapy that are described in manuals, and that have names, and that is a good thing. Therapists learn specific skills and they work within the boundaries of a specific plan. The world needs more of this kind of therapy, provided with the same kind of financial coverage that is available for drug treatments and operations. What may be surprising, however, is that for the most part, although these therapies work, they don't work *because* of their specific targets and principles and activities. These specific elements – the things that are different from one mode of therapy to the next – account for about 15 per cent of the benefits from therapy. A much larger part of the secret sauce, about 30 per cent, is due to what all of these therapies have in common when they are practiced effectively. The common factors are a strong alliance between the therapist and the client, empathy, adjustment in response to feedback from the client, genuineness, positive regard, and the therapist's ability to manage strong emotions. Effective therapists pay attention to those common factors, and that makes a big difference. Clients of effective therapists are twice as likely to get better and half as likely to deteriorate as clients of ineffective therapists, no matter what mode of therapy they are practicing.

Jon picked up the conversation. "The potential for psychotherapy to cause harm is not just for patients. If we are talking about cautionary tales, I think we need to include vicarious trauma to therapists. When you talk about this stuff, you have taken to saying you're 'a little bit broken.'"

I agreed, cautiously. "Yeah, although I feel reluctant to make too great a claim to being traumatized. We're not like war veterans or anything."

"No, but your 'fever' was pretty unsettling. It took some therapy to put the pieces back together."

"And there are changes that linger," I continued. "I think they are permanent but who knows."

"Such as?"

"Well, we've both talked about noticing some signs of burnout creeping in. Being tired of stepping up to be supportive and empathic for yet another person overwhelmed by anxiety or to take the brunt of someone's anger while we help them figure out what is going on. Wanting a little distance. I daydream of retirement. That sort of thing. But I also have more bad dreams than I think I would if I wasn't doing this work. I have an ACE score of zero, but I feel as if I've experienced some terrible things, just by being there to hear about them so many times."

Jon leaned forward. "I had an awful fucking nightmare last week. Stayed with me the whole next day. I can't believe what our patients have to live with. It was terrible."

I continued. "I am aware that I have an exaggerated fear about innocent people being harmed in one way or another – just in the back of my head, a kind of wariness. Also, and it's hard to know if it is related to work at all, but if I'm not thoughtful about it, I'll drink more wine than I should. I feel like I deserve it."

Jon protested gently. "Yeah. But I push back about calling that 'broken.' You're still working fine. So am I. Nothing's broken. It's just wear and tear."

"Which is why I'm reluctant to claim too much. I think someone else would say, 'you're not so special. That's just what happens with experience. It's just life. You're old.'"

"I think it's more than that."

"So maybe 'a little bit broken'?"

Jon smiled. "Fuck off."

Psychotherapy is complicated and taxing and sometimes things catch you by surprise, like "I'd exterminate him." Those are the moments to step back, recognize a misunderstanding or a misstep, ask for help if you need it, refocus on the basics, and get back to work.

16

"Boohoo"

About nine years into therapy, Isaac took a week off. When he came back, he told me that he had gone to Texas on short notice to help a friend. His friend was married and having an affair with a much younger woman, Jen, who was pregnant. Isaac went down to go to the abortion clinic with Jen.

I could feel my reactions brewing up. I didn't know the friend but I had already decided he was an asshole. Isaac's description of Jen, on the other hand, was touching. He was sympathetic and respectful. I tried to imagine the circumstances that would lead Jen to draw on the support of a total stranger. Isaac the fixer. Isaac the protector.

"I feel like something terrible happened, and I was part of it."

"Do you mean the abortion?"

"No. That was what she decided to do. I was just there to help. I have no reservations about abortion. But something terrible happened, and I'm implicated."

Isaac cried. It was perhaps the second time that I had seen him cry, and he couldn't stop. I kept my next patient waiting fifteen minutes as Isaac cried and then calmed himself.

The next week, he mocked his crying almost as soon as he came in and sat down.

"Yeah, let's talk about that. Boohoo. Fuck."

He struggled to be more articulate about what had upset him, using words that are very much like the way he sometimes describes his abuse.

"Something happened but I don't know what it was. I was there. I'm implicated. I don't think she's going to be okay."

I listened and tried to understand. There was nothing more to do than to stay present with him while he was feeling so tender and confused.

Over the next few weeks, knee pain that had been bothering Isaac for a few months intensified until it was intolerable. He said it felt like a spike was sticking through the joint and the bone.

"I want to put a spike through my head. That would be perfect. Nail me to the floor ... I'm not going to be able to walk. It's my right knee. I won't be able to drive."

Isaac started talking about getting an amputation. I think he was serious. I must have looked skeptical or maybe I smiled, thinking he was joking, because he changed the subject to tell a joke.

"So a boy walks in on his parents having wild sex and says, 'What are you doing?' His father says, "Go back to your room for twenty minutes and I'll come tuck you in.' The father goes into his son's room a while later and finds the boy is having wild sex with his grandmother. The father yells, 'What are you doing?' and the kid says, 'See. It's not so funny when it's *your* mother.' That's a psychiatry joke."

I didn't laugh. My facial expression probably conveyed what I was thinking: *What the fuck was* that *for?* He was in pain. My intention was to understand and empathize, but instead we were sparring.

Isaac paused and returned to talking about Jen. Although he hadn't mentioned her in a couple of weeks, he told me that he couldn't get the abortion off his mind. He called it heartbreaking.

I said, "We don't often talk about love, but when you tell me that you are heartbroken, you are lovable. It is a tender, human response to a heartbreaking experience. You don't usually allow yourself that. Just like when you allowed yourself to cry."

Isaac said, "We are not going to meet for a couple of weeks because of the holiday. I feel like we should shake hands." I stood up as Isaac got up to leave and we shook hands. As he left, he said, "You know that is the first time we've ever touched."

When Isaac came back in January, the knee pain was unrelenting. He talked about his inevitable decline and death. He found respite in the idea that he would get a hotel room and take an overdose with fantastic drugs. We talked about the options, and he agreed to go back on an antidepressant drug that he had stopped for a few months.

He couldn't stop thinking about Jen and their visit to the abortion clinic. He wouldn't linger on the feeling long but he acknowledged feeling regret for his role there.

I said, "You know, what comes to mind is that Leonard Cohen line from 'Bird on a Wire': 'Like a baby stillborn, like a beast with his horn, I have torn everyone who reached out for me.'"

"Uh-huh." Isaac paused a few seconds. "I am thinking about how innocent people suffer. That girl, Jen. Kids."

I was thinking about ten-year-old Isaac, but I didn't say anything. He cried again.

"I don't know what I'd do without you, Bob. I don't think I'd be here."

Two weeks later, Isaac returned from a trip to Washington with his wife, Sarah. They traveled there to attend Barack Obama's inauguration. He was beaming. It was hard to walk around in downtown Washington with his knee, but they found a place where they could sit. He told me that the pain was just as severe as ever but more tolerable somehow. He allowed himself to hope.

AS OUR WORK PROGRESSES, Isaac relaxes his defenses at times. The walls go back up afterward, but for a while, he feels safe enough to take some chances. He cries about something heartbreaking and then he hardens up and mocks himself for it. And so it goes, back and forth. As with so many of the experiences that he shares with me, his trip to Texas is not fully explained. I don't really know why he was compelled to help Jen. He was loyal to his friend. I think her situation probably reminded him of others who have been closer to him in the past. I do know that his impulse to protect and support her was a genuine act of love for a relative stranger. It is an important event in Isaac's therapy, so it is worth taking a short diversion into psychological theory to understand why.

Jon and I turn to attachment theory to understand how people use their closest relationships to manage threats and stresses. Although the name makes people think about attachment parenting (skin-to-skin contact at birth and co-sleeping and stuff like that), that is not what we are talking about. It was attachment theory that I was using in Chapter 3 to describe patterns of using interpersonal relationships to manage the feelings that result from early adversity (distance and avoidance, or anxious preoccupation and clinging). The theory was developed by John Bowlby, a child psychoanalyst.

Bowlby was seven at the start of World War I. He had been raised by his nanny for his first four years, having had little contact with his father, the royal surgeon, Major-General Sir Anthony Bowlby, and his emotionally distant mother, Lady May Bowlby. The war was a suitable excuse to send John and his brother to boarding school, "the traditional first step in the time-honored barbarism required to produce an English gentleman." It was a child-rearing tradition that he later said he would not impose on a dog. It is fitting that much later, when Bowlby was the medical director of the Tavistock Clinic in London, which provided psychological care to children and families, he would break with psychoanalytic tradition to insist that actual experiences, rather than just internal mental dynamics, shape individual psychology. Like many revolutionary ideas, once that idea is accepted, in retrospect it seems obvious. That was the seed of attachment theory, which remains profoundly influential. Few other psychological theories are as robustly supported by evidence.

One of Bowlby's insights might help to understand Isaac's motivation for his trip to Texas. Isaac consistently manages feelings of fear, sadness, and shame – the kind of feelings that make a person cry – by keeping those feelings to himself. Instead of allowing himself to look weak or ask for help, he keeps others at bay, often with bravado and hostility. That is an interpersonal style that Bowlby called *compulsive self-reliance*. Of course, Isaac, just like everyone else, needs people. Keeping others at an emotional distance isn't a way of getting rid of them; it is a way of staying in a relationship with them. Keeping connected requires keeping others at a safe distance and appearing to be intact.

But Bowlby also recognized there was a common variant of compulsive self-reliance that he called *compulsive caregiving*. It is a pattern in which people are so engaged in being the supporter of others that their own needs and vulnerabilities barely even register. For many people, compulsive caregiving is a description of most of their close relationships. Often, it is a source of pride. In an early therapy conversation, it can be a turning point when someone who says, "I am the one everyone counts on. I'm a really good listener. I make sure the others are okay," comes to realize how hard it is for them to ask for help for themselves. Some evidence suggests that of all the ways that a person can manage feeling insecure, this way has the best outcomes. Compulsively keeping your troubles to yourself is not ideal, but as one of the ways to manage feelings of insecurity, caregiving might be one of the healthiest.

For Isaac, caregiving in this way is not habitual; it is special. It is probably how he parents a lot of the time, but not how Sarah would describe their relationship. So, an episode like the trip to Texas is a special exception – a brief shift toward a healthier version of his dismissive solution to feeling broken and implicated. In that sense, it fits that the trip to support Jen occurred around the same time that he was prepared to allow himself to cry and, even more specially, to allow himself to hope.

Although the compulsive caregiving solution to perpetually feeling insecure is just one of several possible outcomes of early adversity and invalidation, it is worth a brief diversion, if only because I imagine some readers might recognize themselves in the description. One point to make is that I call it a "solution" intentionally. *Everyone* tries to organize their life and relationships to feel as safe and secure as possible. To get all existential for a second, human beings are virtually defenseless – naked mammals, born helpless, unable to survive their first few years without attaching to a protector *somehow*, perpetually needing others and yet alone in a world whose fundamental meaning and purpose is either opaque or absent and whose inhabitants are routinely indifferent or combative. *Every* solution to the insecurity that state of affairs creates is valuable. Whatever gets you through the night.

So, when I say that the compulsive caregiving style is a defense against insecurity, understand that I do not mean that it would be better to be defenseless. Psychological defenses only become a problem when they are so inflexible that a person cannot adapt to new circumstances or when they are misapplied in situations in which actual risks are low. Psychotherapy is a process of recognizing defenses and sometimes relaxing them, as is happening for Isaac at this point. However, good therapists are careful about that – you don't mess with defenses unless you are sure you have something better to offer. Most people are not inclined to give up their preferred defenses anyway. You are much more likely to find your *partner's* defenses a problem then your own.

For people who are compulsive caregivers, the trouble comes when they actually could use some support from someone else and they don't get it. That hurts and often leads to a painful combination of resentment (for the lack of support) and self-blame (for the inability to ask for it). It is no surprise that the recognition of need or the offer of support is not forthcoming; the relationship is built on the premise that that person is a support provider, not a support needer. These folks often just tough it out, or if they have the good luck to be partnered up with a mind reader, get some of what they need in spite of not asking. Compulsive caregivers make good health care professionals, but their skills don't work as well when they are patients.

As the story of Isaac's time with me shows, psychotherapy is not a journey. Journeys, even circuitous ones, are much too linear to serve as an apt metaphor. But there is an *intention* to change that is relatively linear, progressing from one goal to the next. In the terms of attachment theory, the intention is usually to progress from a position of insecurity to one of greater security – which means greater tolerance of the anxiety of being alone plus greater openness to intimacy with others. That is usually matched by moving toward a position of greater flexibility in expressing emotion – being able to move between open expression and keeping things to yourself as fits the circumstance, rather than being inflexibly stuck in just one of those modes. When Isaac moves from his usual position of maintaining a safe emotional distance through fierce independence and intimidation to one of compassionate care for someone else, he is moving in that direction of intended change. Toward greater flexibility, more open expression of emotion, and greater intimacy. Obama wrote of the audacity of hope. We allowed ourselves a bit of that audacity for a moment.

17

Running

"I was having a shower and felt this lump" is the beginning of a conversation most doctors recognize. It comes with urgency, fear, and uncertainty. The silent communication: "I don't know if this is really a thing or not. I need you to tell me to take this seriously or to relax." It leads quickly to a physical exam – nothing else matters as much as the lump.

Isaac found a lump in his armpit. He knew that the medication he was taking for Crohn's disease can cause lymphoma, so he was worried. He immediately called his family doctor and took the first available appointment, even though he would see a resident instead of Simon, his own doctor. It was better than waiting.

At the appointment, the day after he found the lump, it had already gotten smaller and harder to find. The resident was still training but she knew what she was doing. She reassured Isaac: "Bad things don't go away."

That's where Isaac started when we met the next day.

"'Bad things don't go away.' She doesn't know how right she was about that."

"It's like a one-sentence description of your life: bad things don't go away."

We shared the relief of a lump transformed from the only thing that matters to nothing at all. And then we took a moment to pay attention to his response to the danger sign, which was a timely, appropriate, and effective request to see a doctor.

It wasn't always like that.

When Isaac was twelve, his mother took him on the long bus ride to the doctor their family had been seeing since before he was born. He hadn't been to the doctor for three years. Unless the school insisted on a vaccination, it never seemed like a priority.

His fear grew as they sat on the bus. He was thinking about the young man next door and his threats. If Isaac ever told anyone what the young man did, the man would kill Isaac's mother. Isaac believed the threat, but even worse was the shame and the terror of being discovered, his sense that he was implicated in a terrible act.

He sat silently on the bus thinking that somehow the doctor was going to figure out what had happened to him. *He's going to know. He will know.* He didn't know how the doctor would figure it out, just that somehow it would be obvious to him. *He will know.*

When they got off the bus, his mother turned toward the doctor's office and Isaac took off at full speed in the opposite direction. He was out of his mother's sight in no time at all, and she had no idea where he went. Eventually she just went home.

Isaac didn't return home until late that night. His parents didn't ask him why he had run or where he went. His dad yelled at him. He was in big trouble but he didn't care. The punishment couldn't compare to the shame averted.

He didn't see another doctor until he had his first operation a decade later.

About four years later, Isaac needed braces. That's what the dentist said, so his parents sent him to an orthodontist. He lay back in the chair. He was used to the routine, but the orthodontist was new to him so Isaac was wary, checking out the scene. Isaac always knows where the exits are.

The orthodontist said nothing but "open your mouth." Isaac opened his mouth and the man put something into it – a piece of equipment, his fingers, an instrument – Isaac had no idea. Whatever it was, it felt shocking, unexpected, overpowering.

Maybe it was something in the man's manner or the command. Maybe it was something about the feel of the thing in his mouth. Isaac still can't figure it out. Almost fifty years later he still gets anxious telling the story.

He jumped from the orthodontist's chair and ran from the office. They were probably yelling at him as he left. It's all a blur. Isaac didn't see another dentist until he was thirty.

A year or two after starting therapy, Isaac was preparing for surgery. Another resection, another foot of scarred and twisted bowel needed to be removed.

At the pre-op clinic, swabs were required to see if he carried any bacteria that would put other patients at risk. The nurse did not explain this. She just said, "I'm going to stick this up your nose."

"The fuck you are. Give it to me. I'll do it."

The next swab was of the skin in the crack of his buttocks. The nurse said, "Drop your pants."

Isaac said, "Stick it up your own ass," and left. Once again, he was "a difficult patient." At times like that you can't see his fear through its thick veil of anger.

The recent story of the-lump-that-went-away is an excellent exception to a lifetime of running away from health care. Isaac has worked hard to achieve it. He needed help, asked for it, and help was given. As an extra bonus, something bad appeared, and then it went away. Excellent exceptions are the footholds of change.

ASKING FOR HELP CAN be an achievement. Sometimes the difficulty is obvious, as in Isaac's doomed attempts in Chapter 14 (the note, the smashed bicycle, the prescription). Sometimes it is more subtle, as for a compulsive caregiver (Chapter 16), who always finds someone else's needs to be more urgent. It may seem like too simple a point to belabor, but our health care system is built for people who show up, identify a problem, and ask for help. It works well for a person who does what Isaac did with his lump.

His timely and appropriate call led to the reassurance that he needed about as quickly as can happen. But it isn't always like that.

Adults with childhood experiences like Isaac's often have similar problems attending a family doctor or a dentist. Amelia was a patient of mine for even longer than Isaac. She went over twenty years without seeing a dentist in spite of increasingly painful problems with her teeth. She had tried to go a long time earlier but her panic once she got in the dentist's chair was too intense to bear. It was, as for Isaac, connected to specific traumatic memories connected to her mouth. The reasons for fear are not always so specific (dental phobias are pretty common), but you don't know the source of someone else's fear unless you ask. In the end, Amelia was able to overcome her fear and get the dental care she needed by collaborating with a skilled and extraordinarily patient dentist who worked through the fear with her by giving her lots of time, clear communication, and control over the process as much as possible – by agreeing on signals to stop the work or by having sessions where she sat in the chair while no work was done, so she could wait out the fear without fleeing. Amelia's dentist was amazing, but also exceptional; our health care system is not equipped to provide that kind of care. We are too focused on supposed efficiency ("supposed" because there is no actual efficiency in providing ineffective care or excluding those who can't accommodate) and on the technical, rather than relational, aspects of our work. For the most part, the system fails to even recognize that it needs to accommodate people like Amelia.

Going to the doctor involves many things that a person like Isaac prefers to avoid – answering questions, exposing his body, allowing himself to be touched, and allowing someone else to make decisions that determine how he feels. It involves transactions that are predicated on tolerating vulnerability, trust, and negotiating authority over one's body. Going to the doctor often involves having something stuck in you – a needle, a finger, a speculum, a tongue depressor. We call those acts *invasive*, which is accurate, but also technical enough to distance ourselves a little bit from the ones getting stuck. Isaac tries to bridge that distance: "Stick it up your own ass."

How patients deal with the intrusion affects their health. Take, for example, early detection of prostate cancer in men, which requires checking on the prostate from time to time when it isn't causing any problems. There are two ways to check: a digital rectal exam (finger in the anus) and a blood test (PSA, a protein that is released from the prostate into the bloodstream when the cells are cancerous). Both tests are somewhat invasive. Men who are dismissing and self-reliant, like Isaac, have each of these tests less often than other men. Same thing for women regarding breast self-examination and mammograms. The result can only be that cancer prevention is more effective for those with low ACE scores. Another line of dominoes in the story of child maltreatment as a cause of causes of disease and early mortality.

Something similar happens for people with diabetes, one of the most common and consequential chronic diseases. People with diabetes get a lot of education about managing the disease, because it is complicated to eat and exercise in a way that keeps blood sugar under control, and much more complicated once control of the disease requires treatment with insulin injections or an insulin pump. Diabetes education programs are an exemplar of efforts to facilitate self-management and patient-centered care. Diabetes educator is a job that has specific training requirements and certification. There are not many diseases for which there is an actual job named "[insert disease name here] educator."

One of the results of diabetes education is that people with the disease know to pay attention to their HbA1c (glycated hemoglobin). It is a blood test that summarizes how well they have controlled their blood sugar levels over the previous three months. People who find numbers helpful focus their diabetic care on reducing HbA1c. People with Isaac's interpersonal style, dismissing, self-reliant, distancing people, have substantially higher HbA1c than all others, in the high range that is associated with the grave complications of poorly controlled disease – *if* they have a poor relationship with their diabetes doctor, but not otherwise.

Imagine what is going on there. Two Isaacs show up at the diabetes clinic. They are hard to engage. They don't like monitoring their blood sugar levels several times a day. Being self-reliant, they think that managing their diet and activity the way they want to makes more sense than doing what the educator says. Insulin gives them a powerful tool to influence their health and how they feel. At first, their plan doesn't go well: blood sugar tests show levels that are all over the map and HbA1c rises. Our two Isaacs have different doctors. The first one reacts by doubling down, insisting on more blood tests, more frequent visits to the clinic, stricter adherence to diet. He doesn't read the interpersonal clues; he scolds and blames. So, Isaac doesn't come back. He looks angry but he feels humiliated. The second doctor finds a different path. She tries to find a way to meet Isaac where he is. She asks him about his goals and what is working and not working in their effort to meet them. She doesn't assume that her goals (including an all-star HbA1c) are his. They figure out how to muddle through, together. (The doctors' gender is irrelevant. One is a man and one a woman to keep them straight here.)

When doctors were interviewed about challenging situations in which their goals and their patients' goals don't align, they emphasized the effort that they make to get on the same page. One said, "There's a ton of negotiation that goes on ... Half of what we do is trying to understand what the patient's real concerns are, what they would like to have done or what they expect would be done and then negotiating something sensible at the end of it." Another said, "It's not necessarily a short-term goal [that matters most] ... all the encounters are to come to some sort of agreement about what we're doing ... so there's consensus between both myself and the patient that this is what we want to work toward. But for some of these patients and symptoms, that could take a very long time to come to."

It is obvious to those who are poorly served that the health care system has built-in barriers, whether they are disadvantaged by being uninsured, addicted, inarticulate, unable to speak the dominant language, disabled, mentally ill, or targets of stigma and discrimination for reasons of skin color, sexuality, culture, or gender. The point that we are making with the stories of Isaac's running stands in addition to those – the system doesn't serve those who don't show up. Those who don't show up are disproportionately the survivors of childhood maltreatment. When they do show up, we who are within the system have a responsibility to not do things that make them want to flee.

Doctors express their frustration at patients who don't accept their advice by choosing words like *noncompliance* and *rejecting help* (and typically don't give a second thought to people who don't show up at all). For the millions whose health care interactions are shaped by childhood adversity, those words miss the point; the fundamental problem is not stubbornness or hostility – it is fear. And fear has to be met with patience, respect, and empathy.

18

"Who is going to give a shit?"

Isaac has needed surgery every six or seven years. In the intervening years, his symptoms don't subside completely, and he has often been in the position of seeing a surgeon, not knowing if they will think it is time for another operation, and not knowing whether to wish for that as a source of relief or to dread it. It was at a time like that, in those intervening years, that Isaac was sitting in the office of Joan, his surgeon. She looked intently at her computer screen, clicking slowly through the hundreds of frames of a CT scan of his abdomen. She had the radiologist's report, but now she was rechecking for herself. Joan looked up. "I can't operate. There's nothing here for me to fix. It all looks pretty good. The wall of the small bowel is a little thick in one place. I can't tell if it is inflammation or scarring, but it is not enough to cause the pain you've got."

"You don't know how much this hurts. I can't eat anything."

"I can't keep prescribing Percocet. You don't need a surgeon right now, so I can't keep giving you these painkillers."

"What am I supposed to do? I can't live like this."

Isaac left her office feeling angry and entirely alone. There was no point seeing his gastroenterologist. Nothing had changed since that specialist had told Isaac that his inflammation was well enough controlled and that he would never prescribe pain medication. Within the silos of their specialties, neither of the experts was wrong. Isaac didn't have what they were experts at treating. He understood that, but it didn't matter.

"What am I supposed to do? Who is going to give a shit about me? I can't eat because of the pain."

He found a solution. He spoke to Simon, his family doctor, who agreed to prescribe a safe dose of the pain medication and to closely monitor how Isaac was using the pills. This required compromises by Simon, who would prefer to treat the pain without this medication, and by Isaac, who agreed to tolerate closer monitoring than he prefers. It was a compromise that fits with the idea of harm reduction – the prescription plan isn't ideal, but refusing it is likely to put Isaac at risk of greater harm. I didn't broker the deal, but I was with Isaac, at least in his mind, while he sorted it out.

Isaac's surgeon and his gastroenterologist are good doctors, and they care about their patients. Each has advocated to Jon or me on a patient's behalf at different times. We can't blame the problem with Isaac's health care on bad apples in the profession. Indeed, a great deal of what is wrong with health care is not the fault of the professionals or the patients. It is how we have lost sight of the importance of the relationships between them.

KAREN LE AND I have worked together for a decade since she first came to the hospital to do her master's degree. She is Dr. Le now and has led a series of studies that trace a path from early adversity to insecure attachment relationships to risky behaviors like smoking and excessive drinking. After a few years away, she came back to the hospital to develop a deeper understanding of how early relationships influence the way patients experience physical symptoms and health worries. She interviewed patients who struggle with symptoms, as Isaac does, or with health anxiety and she talked to their family doctors. Although Karen chose patients to interview based on their problems with physical symptoms – they weren't selected for having childhood adversity – most had elevated ACE scores.

There were no surprises in what the patients and doctors identified as contentious situations. They each identified that it caused problems when a patient wants a medication but the doctor isn't thrilled about it (usually pain medication) or when a doctor wants to prescribe a medication but the patient isn't thrilled about it (usually psychiatric medication). Disagreements about the cause of symptoms were common, typically that patients think the source is physical while doctors think that it is psychological. Another common source of contention was when patients want tests to investigate their symptoms while doctors prefer to avoid them. They were both worried that some serious disease would be missed because its symptoms had been attributed to anxiety. Good doctors worry about this *a lot*. At their worst, the tensions can end the relationship; patients spoke of walking out and of threatening lawsuits, doctors of being relieved when they were "fired." What was especially compelling, though, was what they had to say about how they worked through the tension.

Both patients and doctors emphasized the value of listening well, feeling validated, negotiating a consensus, and finding ways to agree on goals. Bad experiences that were recalled often were the result of poor listening, or a closed mind that felt like it silenced or invalidated the patient's perspective. For example, a patient who had an ACE score of seven recalled a visit with a doctor in which "it was a very one-way kind of thing. And I honestly walked out, because she wasn't listening ... everything was, like, pills shoved down my throat, that's the solution. But I'm, like, telling her ... I'm getting therapy, I'm reading books, I'm trying to practice mindfulness. I don't think pills are the only solution here."

Relationships between patients and health care professionals are built on collaboration. The therapeutic alliance between a patient and a health care provider consists of three things: a relationship of sufficient trust, agreement on goals, and agreement on strategies to reach those goals. Without that alliance, care is barely possible. The patients and doctors that Karen Le interviewed described a lot of negotiating to agree on goals and how to reach them. Their opening negotiating positions could be quite far apart. One patient (ACE score of four) needed control over a diet that doctors thought was unhealthy: "My diet is probably bad, but it's good for me because I'm controlling my whole diet and exercise to a science." A different patient and her doctor could agree the goal was to control symptoms but disagreed on strategy. Others had to negotiate to even agree on their goal. A doctor spoke about a patient who continued to look for an elusive cure: "She's like 'once we get this cured I'm going to be back to normal.' And I think, *You've been this way for five years and unfortunately you haven't been able to return to work* ... I don't want to be discouraging but at the same time I want to ... allow them to function as well as they can." When the treatment relationship is strong, they sort it out – or, more likely, it is sorting it out that strengthens the treatment relationship.

A further aspect of an effective collaboration that patients and doctors described was respecting each other's expertise. Patients are experts about their own lives. Doctors are experts about medicine. Each wants to be recognized as such, and the relationship works better when that happens. A patient who had an ACE score of six expressed it clearly. He described that one thing that improves the interactions with doctors "is actually respecting me as a human being, respecting me as somebody who is an equal and knows my problems better than you do, because you're not living it."

Doctors noted the tension that arises when accommodating a patient's wishes would lead to forfeiting their expertise and compromising their professionalism. One told Dr. Le about the "tension of wanting to preserve the doctor-patient relationship but not being prepared to do things or behave in ways that compromise your own sense of professional self."

They are difficult conversations. The interviews revealed that there is often a great deal of good will on both sides of a collaboration, as doctor and patient negotiate a shared understanding of what the problem is and how to manage it. But good will alone is not enough to resolve the inherent tensions. Conversations are complicated because the patients are sometimes reluctant to say what they want. Feeling safe in an interaction like this usually trumps all other considerations. If it doesn't feel emotionally safe to state what you need, it won't happen. A patient who has an ACE score of two reported she would be "too embarrassed to ... say 'I'm frightened of this medication or the impact that this mental illness is having on me, and I need reassurance.' There's no way I would ever do that, it would be humiliating ... I don't know if this is a reasonable expectation, but a good outcome of that would be to feel someone recognizing, acknowledging that, and reassuring me." Intuiting that a patient needs reassurance but is too embarrassed to ask for it is a tall order, especially in a busy clinic with a full waiting room.

Modern health care has all but lost sight of how critical the relationship between health care providers and patients is for care, healing, and prevention. It is the context in which a story that has been fractured by fear can be restored to coherence and the container within which intolerable emotions can resolve into understandable ones. The change that the health care system requires to provide better care to patients like Isaac includes a restoration of the centrality of the relationship between health care providers and patients.

That means promoting health care relationships that are continuous over time, so patient and provider come to know each other; where providers listen more and interrupt less, and where the goal of most health care interactions becomes helping patients with their problems – which is a very different goal than diagnosing and treating their diseases, different enough to be revolutionary.

19

"I've got this figured out"

A couple of years later, Isaac was back in the phase of disease in which surgery was becoming inevitable. The scars that grip his chronically inflamed intestine were gaining too tight a hold. Painful bowel obstructions had always come and gone but now were coming more frequently. He was much less sanguine about the inevitability of another operation then he was when we first met.

"It gets worse every time. I don't know if I can do this again."

"Do you mean the pain?"

"Yes. But no. It's more than that. I think I'm going to die on the table."

I wondered if this was a sign of progress in a weird way. Isaac has never been afraid of dying, so this was a shift – to a fear that is more like what anybody else who was contemplating major surgery might feel. But then he went on.

"I can't get used to the idea of the operating room. What's going to happen?"

"You've been through this so many times. Is there something in particular that's bothering you?"

"It's what I don't know. What do they really do there?"

"What do you mean?"

"Do they tie you down? Do they talk about you?"

"Is that what you've been thinking about?"

"I had a dream."

Isaac stopped speaking for a few minutes while he found the right words or gathered his courage. I just waited for him.

"Joan walks into the operating room."

"This is your dream now?"

He nodded. Joan has been the surgeon for his last couple of operations. He likes her, but more importantly he trusts her expertise. "She walks in, but it isn't Joan. She has this weird crazy look on her face, really menacing. I'm tied down. I can't do anything. Then she gets out the blade – no anesthetic, nobody is ready – and she cuts me open from top to bottom."

Isaac stopped again and gathered his words. "From out of the hole ... from inside me, he comes out. He's huge." Isaac named the young man next door, his abuser for so many years as a boy. "And he says, 'Now you're all going to die.'"

We talked about his dream for a while, getting the details right. The ending obviously had him rattled. It was like a jump cut in a scary movie – the sudden, threatening change that makes you scream.

Over the next couple of weeks, we talked about how to manage these fears. The surgery was inevitable, but maybe it could be easier. Isaac's fearful anticipation of "what really happens" in an operating room remained a preoccupation, so I asked if he wanted to talk to the surgeon about it. I would see if it could be arranged.

He was grateful for the offer but declined. It felt safer to keep his fears to himself. But a week later when I offered again, he said yes. His surgeon was great. They spoke on the phone, and she led him through everything that was likely to happen. He trusted her and felt reassured for a while.

Encouraged by the conversation with Joan, Isaac agreed to talk to the anesthetist about how his pain would be managed, which was also keeping him awake at night. She was practical and realistically reassuring. Once again, Isaac felt that he was in good hands.

One week before surgery, the confidence that Isaac had found started to unravel. A new version of the dream was back, and he couldn't bring himself to talk about it. He was considering calling off the operation, in spite of the pain.

And then, something changed.

"I've got this figured out."

"How?"

"I was thinking about your voice. I can conjure up your voice whenever I want. We've been doing this for so long that you're always with me. What I'm going to do is that I am going to think about that dream image with Joan looking all crazy like the Joker. I'm going to think about it as they wheel me into the operating room. But just as an image, not the whole dream. So, nothing will change, it will just be that image, and then you are going to talk to me."

"What am I going to say?"

"It's not real."

It was a brilliant strategy. Isaac was going to take a dream that was beyond his control and turn it into a still image that he could master – a scary image, but a predictable one. And then he was going to use a relationship that he trusts – the memory of a relationship that he trusts – for solace and protection.

"Do you want me to actually say it? So that it is right in your memory?"

Isaac didn't say anything, but he looked me in the eye and I proceeded.

"It's not real."

Something broke. Isaac wept.

A week later he had his surgery. It was complicated, as hospital stays and operations often are, but he got through it. The last thing he told me before he insisted on leaving hospital, a couple of days before he was really ready, was that we would have to talk about the crying.

"That phrase, 'It's not real' ... it's complicated. I haven't sorted it out yet. But we need to talk about it."

Another step forward.

ISAAC FIGURED OUT A STRATEGY, but imagine what surgery is like for someone who has not been working on the solution for twenty years. How is someone like Isaac supposed to have an operation that he needs while imagining that his tormentor is going to climb out of his belly to wreak havoc again? How is his surgeon supposed to have the first clue that he is even struggling with it?

Trying to answer those questions brings us to *trauma-informed care*. Starting from the work of Dr. Maxine Harris and Dr. Roger Fallot, working around the same time as Felitti's group were producing the ACE study, the movement to make health care services sensitive to how interpersonal violence affects an individual's life has mostly focused on mental health and addiction services. There has been less uptake in medical primary care and virtually none in medical specialties. It is time for change.

Trauma-informed care attends to many kinds of violence and trauma, well beyond childhood adversity, but it also applies to our specific focus. Indeed, disturbingly, often the adults that were exposed to childhood maltreatment and those who have experienced adult trauma are the same people. Trauma-informed care emphasizes strengths over deficits, is attentive to the likelihood that those seeking care have experienced trauma, strives to avoid repeating the trauma, and is directed toward recovery. A health care organization that takes trauma seriously makes sure that every member of its team, from the first contact at the reception desk to the CEO, understands how trauma influences their patients so that every relationship is attentive to enhancing recovery and avoiding re-traumatization.

Here are some principles that health care organizations can adopt:

- Recognize that interpersonal violence influences many parts of a person's being, from personal identity to a survivor's tenuous sense of safety and hope. Therefore, it influences how they cope – especially the likelihood that they will cope by avoiding health care. Recognizing this impact is validating because it allows avoidance to be understood rather than criticized.
- Respect every person's need for safety, respect, and acceptance. Everyone needs to feel safe, but no one quite does. There is virtually

nothing that can be accomplished in health care without first ensuring that a patient feels safe, or at least close enough to safe.

- Empower patients. Help survivors of trauma take charge of their lives and their health care. Maximize their options and their influence. This extends to how the organization conceives of, delivers, and evaluates trauma-informed care. "Nothing about me without me" is a rallying cry of patient-centered care in general. As we saw in Chapter 18, this empowerment emerges from relationships in which the provider and patient respect each other's expertise and work on shared goals that are established collaboratively, and in which patients feel their experiences and choices are validated.

- Appreciate that healing, and all health care, occurs in relationships. Promote continuity (seeing the same health care professional each time) and a strong treatment alliance (trust, shared goals, and agreement on strategies) over the illusion of efficiency. "Illusion" because if services are designed to maximize their apparent efficiency to the organization (for example, by frequently rotating the doctors who are on service because it is convenient to do so) and yet result in costly, repetitive investigations, poor outcomes, and chronic symptoms, where is the actual efficiency?

- Know that the power hierarchy in treatment relationships is inevitable and requires thoughtful consideration. Pretending that Isaac and I are on equal terms in our long, strange dance would be delusional. On one hand, my ability to help requires me to approach the relationship as an expert. On the other hand, Isaac and I must both bear in mind the harms that our power differential can perpetuate. If I were to resolve the discomfort of sharing Isaac's turmoil by reducing him to the subject of my expertise (enacting the hidden curriculum of "us and them" that Jon and I learned in medical school), I would repeat his oppression, literally his subjugation.

- Emphasize patients' strengths rather than their pathology. Highlight successful adaptation rather than symptoms. Some say, "Don't ask *what's wrong with you? Ask what happened to you?*" This principle takes that idea a step further. Don't just ask what happened, also notice that a patient has shown strength in adapting to what happened – even if the adaptations turned into problems over time. Part of helping Isaac come to terms with his smoking was to acknowledge (even admire) how he ingeniously solved an overwhelming threat under the pressure of time and terror when he was eleven years old.

• Minimize re-traumatization. So much of what we do in medicine has the potential to repeat an old trauma. We ask people to get naked; we stick things in them and hurt them. We use our power without asking at times. Avoiding this takes a couple of extra steps, such as when we invite a partner to be present during an exam if wanted, explain a procedure in plain language, and make sure it is okay to proceed, but often those extra steps are all that are required to reduce unnecessary harm.

• Be culturally competent. Understand each patient in the context of their life experiences and background. This is an extension of empathy, in a sense. The role of a health care professional is not to interpret a patient's words or actions through the biases of their own culture and experience but to try to see what it is like from the patient's perspective, through the lens of the patient's own experience and beliefs.

These principles may seem obvious. They may just seem like decent, respectful, empowering care, but they are revolutionary. The revolution wrests power from well-intentioned autocrats, like me, to force a collaboration that values my skills but defers to someone else's perspective. No one who is used to holding power should expect the revolution to be comfortable. If there is one thing that I have learned in working with Isaac and others like him, it is that over-valuing my own comfort is an impediment. Trauma-informed care gives me a road map for valuing respectful, safe care over my comfort.

Sometimes trauma-informed care involves actually asking patients about their experiences so that it is possible to appreciate the circumstances. It needn't always. Instead, a trauma-informed organization can adopt a set of principles to apply to everybody, knowing that there are many patients for whom it is critical and that it isn't practical to try to figure out which those are. This idea of *universal precautions* is the same as how in medicine we assume all blood samples contain something contagious, even though most don't. It is just safer for everyone that way.

My work with Isaac has followed several of the principles of trauma-informed care. Our work has obviously been attentive to his traumatic experiences from the beginning. He has also made sure, starting on that first day, that I see his strengths first and his vulnerabilities only in that context. Neither of us would use the word *recovery* as a goal, but I guess it is true – we are aiming for him feeling more whole and less broken. It is engrained in my psychotherapy training to emphasize the positive adaptations in his responses to trauma, even when the results also cause him further injuries (the smoking, the drugs, his bravado). On the other hand, I have focused on Isaac's deficits deliberately and consistently, often at his insistence. Empathy demands that I have recognized his view of himself, and often its accuracy, as we try to find an alternative perspective.

I think it also matters that I am telling *Isaac's* story. The trauma-informed perspective would favor hearing his voice. However, the alternative to my storytelling is silence or a story shared only between two. "I'm not going to make it. I need you to speak for me" was his instruction to share the power of storytelling. I am doing my best to live up to the bargain.

20

"I used to think that nothing could change"

Back in my office after his surgery, Isaac and I are talking about his slow recovery. He pauses.

"I had a dream that we were talking about that other dream."

"The one from before surgery ..."

"Yeah. In this dream you were telling me that I need to think about it harder. So I've been thinking about it. And the crying."

"Uh-huh."

"And what I came up with is ... It wasn't my fault."

"I don't think you've said that before."

"No. In some ways it doesn't change anything. But it sort of changes everything. I have always known that I have something inside me that is contagious, something that is evil for everyone ... But it's not my fault."

"That feels pretty huge."

"I don't know ... and um, um ... I haven't smoked since the surgery."

"No shit?!"

"I thought ... I started to smoke when I was eleven so no one would know what had happened. I thought they would smell what had happened, and I had to hide it ... And now I think, it wasn't my fault. Fuck that. I don't want to smoke."

"Wow. And it's been a month."

"Yeah. Of course, I'm addicted to nicotine, so I don't know, but right now I think fuck that."

I STARTED TO TELL Isaac's story because I was pissed off that his experience is so common and yet invisible and silent, that it has damaged him for his entire life and was entirely preventable. We have spent twenty years trying to heal this harm, and we're not done yet. I don't know if Isaac will ever be healed, but I feel hopeful about how things are changing. I feel more optimistic now than I used to be that Isaac's grandchildren will grow up remembering him and valuing the memories.

The particulars of Isaac's story have led us along a path that is anything but linear, often without fully understanding what we were discussing as it emerged, and sometimes with a sense of apprehension that something even worse was lurking behind the murk. Beyond the particulars, themes emerge that apply to many people who live with the consequences of childhood abuse and adversity.

Here is what Jon and I have learned in thirty years of providing psychiatric care for hundreds of Isaacs since we graduated without a clue.

The person who most needs understanding is the least likely to be understood. What you see is not what you get. Everyone has a story, and if you don't know the story you are likely to misconstrue words, feelings, and actions. You won't see the fear that lies behind their anger, for instance. Or you'll interpret their distance as arrogance rather than shame.

The person most at risk of illness and harm is the least equipped to provide self-care. A person needs to feel safe above all else. A person under threat will do just about anything to feel safer. Sometimes those actions are unhealthy and self-destructive, as illustrated by some of the things Isaac has done to feel safe: smoking, using lots of drugs, running away from home, arguing, keeping a baseball bat under the bed, and refusing hospital care. You need to know a person and their story to see how they are using their strengths to protect themselves.

The person who most needs a relationship is most afraid of it. Healing emerges out of relationships. It might be a partner or a therapist, a family member, a sponsor, or someone else. But healing from trauma requires a relationship. It makes sense; the harm that was done almost always occurred within a relationship, usually in violation of all of the safety and respect that the relationship was supposed to provide.

Learning to trust, to share, to care, is sometimes a bridge too far for a survivor of trauma. Sometimes it requires more than a partner or therapist can offer. Indeed, Isaac's story illustrates that when a therapist accepts that responsibility, it comes with a risk of getting caught in friendly fire. The same is true for partners, family members, and friends. But when healing occurs, it usually happens within relationships that are reliable enough, tolerant enough, and supportive enough: good enough.

HEALING AND PREVENTION REQUIRE that we open our eyes to what is right before us and that we tell the truth about it. We don't need any more evidence about how common childhood abuse and other forms of adverse experiences are. We don't need to prove that these experiences affect well-being throughout life. We need change.

To see childhood harm for what it is means to be immersed in it, at least a little bit, at least for a while. It also means considering the possibility that there is no division between "us" and "them." It means re-evaluating the spanking or shouting or touching that you may have seen or experienced or done.

As we have argued elsewhere, adverse childhood experiences "are not a black mark that distinguishes between good parents and bad parents. They don't emerge, usually, from malevolent hearts. To end the cycle, we need to change the environment in which families operate. The changes that are required are big: effective treatment for mental illness and addiction, livable incomes, support for parents who need to work and parents who need to stay home, well-resourced day care, education that helps parents to tune into a child's world and respond with sensitivity."

There are far too many people like Isaac who suffer the effects of childhood abuse, neglect, and adversity. Let's summon the courage and humility to accept that we are all a little bit broken, and recognize the power that emerges between people who work to respect, understand, and care for each other. Let's be pissed off together. Let's take a lesson from Isaac and say that we used to think that nothing could change, but now we think *fuck that*.

21

The Care Revolution

Health care needs fixing. Healing is broken when it fails to recognize an extremely common cause of illness and fails to employ one of its most effective tools to promote recovery: safe, respectful, and understanding care relationships. Specialists, who are really partialists, need to have collaborative, caring relationships with whole people. Patients need to be empowered to be full partners in those relationships. We shouldn't aim to change Isaac to fit the world; we need to change the world.

Society needs fixing too. We have all the evidence we need that the maltreatment of children like Isaac causes lifelong damage and is enormously costly in both human and economic terms. And yet, it is preventable. We have stacks of reports, guidelines, and road maps produced by the experts around the world that say very similar things about the social changes needed to prevent maltreatment in the first place.

The solution, in each case, is found in relationships – especially between health care providers and patients, and within families. Parents and everyone else who cares for kids – grandparents, teachers, early childhood educators, foster parents, the whole lot – need support. Not pressure to be perfect, but support to be good enough as they do the hard work of tuning in to and responding to their kids' changing needs as they grow.

So, we know what is wrong, and we think we know how to fix it. What we need is the will to make changes that are revolutionary because they shift the balance of power between patients, generalist health care providers, and specialists. And revolutionary because they shift the balance of cultural values from the autonomy of parents to the human rights of children, because they take society's investment in fixing broken adults and put it toward raising strong children, to paraphrase Frederick Douglass.

As Jon and I learned in our early years of practice, the revolution demands that we open our eyes to what is actually in front of us instead of seeing what we expect or what we wish. And as with every revolution, change demands that we all feel and respect the unease that is inevitable when we allow ourselves to fully appreciate our current state, in which kids are maltreated and damaged for life while most of us look the other way. The revolution demands that we do what is right instead of what is easy.

This is not a violent revolution; it is a revolution of *care*. Compassion. Respect. Empathy. Validation. Collaboration. Honesty.

What can be done? Lots. What follows is our prescription to make relationships of care central to health, health care, and society, addressed to those whose roles are crucial: Health care providers, their students, health care and child welfare organizations, parents, citizens, and patients. When the topic is health care providers, we'll stay in our lane to talk about doctors, the group Jon and I know best. We encourage our colleagues in other disciplines of health care to turn their spotlight on their own groups.

Doctors

Jon and I are standing on a stage in front of a room of a couple of hundred family doctors, who have taken time away from their busy practices to attend an educational conference. We've done the formal part of our talk. I have presented the evidence linking ACEs to their patients' most common medical problems and making clear how many of their patients have high ACE scores. Jon has described the CARE method of asking about childhood adversity (see the box on page 164). We have some time for discussion. Several hands go up.

Jon points to someone near the front, who starts things off. "I'm convinced about the relationship between adversity and illness. We see that all the time with our patients. But I don't see the point in asking people who are coming to see me, say, to treat high blood pressure – asking them about what happened when they were kids. It would feel incongruous, and what am I supposed to do with the information anyway?"

"Thanks for this," Jon replies. "It's a great starting point. This goes to the issue of building an alliance with your patient. The main point is that ACEs affect your patient's capacity to participate in hypertension treatment, taking medication regularly or sticking to a program of diet or exercise or whatever, so it isn't different from hypertension treatment; it is part of it. Their treatment will go better if you have a strong relationship. Besides, if they don't have any of these experiences, a negative answer takes less than a minute of time, and if positive, it is still only a couple of minutes to identify a risk factor for many ailments, way beyond their blood pressure.

"Don't get me wrong," Jon continues, "the difficulty with introducing the topic is real; we get that. We have heard it from lots of our colleagues. It sounds like you need some hints about how to link the inquiry to the health management piece so it doesn't feel so incongruous. That's what the CARE method is about."

A doctor a few rows back doesn't wait to be called upon. She stands up, looking annoyed. "I have ten minutes with a patient. Fifteen if I push it, but the waiting room is full. The patient has a specific question for me – maybe we need to adjust medication for arthritis, or they have some new symptom that needs investigation – I can't possibly add an extra conversation to that appointment, even if it 'only takes five minutes' like you say, which I doubt. Do the math. I've got twelve hundred patients. I don't have that many hours. I'm already working sixty hours a week."

I take a breath to respond and am relieved when Jon beats me to it. "Bob and I are not primary care docs. We don't know what we don't know. So, for sure, tell us. There may well be an impossibility to doing it at a time like that. But you do schedule different types of appointments, right? You would take more time to do a Pap smear or to do the history and physical for a new patient. This inquiry probably fits better into a time like that, which is less targeted on a specific question and is already taking a big picture approach. Pick your spots, maybe?"

I don't think we are going to convince this doctor, but I add a bit that may help the rest of the audience. "If I can just add a point about the math. This is not a conversation that you are going to have every appointment. It is like finding out about allergies or a family history of something. Once you know, you know – it will only come up when it matters after that."

A younger doctor has had her hand up for a while. I invite her to speak. "While you were talking, I was thinking about a patient who is often on my mind. I've been seeing her for a few years, since she was in university. She has lots of physical problems – the details probably don't matter. The thing is that I never felt like I was getting anywhere with her. She would always come for her appointments and we would treat this problem and then that problem, but I felt like I was missing something and her quality of life was poor – living by herself and just holding on to a job that was hard and didn't pay much. I felt like I was not giving her what she needed, but I really didn't know. It was just a feeling. And then one day, I just decided to ask her about this stuff. I don't think I said *trauma*. But I had been reading about these things. And I said, 'Let's make another appointment to deal with the symptoms you've got now. For today, can I just ask you about your life? Because sometimes people have experienced bad things, and it affects their physical health. I just wonder if you have lived through things that I should know about' ... And it changed everything. We talked for maybe a half hour. She told me about really difficult circumstances when she was a teenager and how she got away from it and went to university. We haven't talked about it much more since, but that conversation has really changed the feeling when we meet. I don't think it was the information that changed things for me. I don't know if I make decisions differently than I would otherwise. But our relationship is completely different. I think I'm helping her now."

The doctor who asked the time question frowns and shakes her head at the mention of a half hour. Jon responds to the young doctor. "Well, thank you for that. This is the kind of outcome that can happen. *Yes*, it did take longer, and probably stalled your office for that thirty minutes."

"It was the end of the day. That was part of what freed me up to ask a different question."

"Okay, that makes sense. And it was apparently a non sequitur, so it would feel like a leap. But actually, the point is that it was entirely on target. When you were doing the so-called regular appointments, nothing good was happening. You were both frustrated by the lack of resolution and locked into a repetitive, unproductive style of meetings ... this was the time when you got to what mattered. It is like realizing that a rash is never going to go away no matter how much cortisone you slather on it, until the person stops eating gluten. It got you to the heart of an issue that needed attention, and not getting at the cause was never going to be sufficient. It may feel like a risk to take that time, but we have heard this story before ..."

"And you were actually *increasing* your efficiency. Wasting time with short appointments that don't help is false efficiency." I finish Jon's sentence for him.

He looks over at me, smiles, and takes the discussion back. "Your point is not about efficiency though. Your analysis of this patient's situation was spot on, I think. I would even say that it wasn't really the content of what she told you that mattered – what her bad experiences were – it was her experience of you as a concerned, 'cares enough to figure her out' kind of doctor that mattered. One aspect of most ACEs is that the people who should've cared for her didn't, for whatever reason. By disrupting your day to see what is really going on with her, you are like the mother who sees her kid isn't sleeping and instead of just closing the door because she is pooped from a long day asks the kid what is wrong and finds out they are being bullied at school."

Jon points toward a serious-looking man with his hand up: "You guys are researchers. So, you know about test characteristics. Asking about

ACEs is a screening test. If you ask people who are likely to give a positive answer, then it may be a good test – the response will be meaningful. But if you ask everyone, your rate of false positives is going to be high. And you have nothing to do for people who have answered positively. So, you are creating anxiety for no purpose. I think it is unethical."

I take this one. "That is a technical point as well as an ethical one. I'll remind the others in the room who need a refresher on test characteristics that, as you know, every diagnostic test is falsely positive sometimes. In people who are likely to have what you are testing for, a positive test is more likely to be true. If you test only people who are unlikely to have a diagnosis, then most of your positives are false positives. But here's the thing. Asking about ACEs *is not* a diagnostic test. Having experienced adversity is not a diagnosis. It is your patient's history – like asking about allergies. You don't wait until you are suspicious to ask; you ask everyone, mostly so you won't inadvertently harm them.

"And to be clear, we are not advocating giving your patients the ACE questionnaire. We are advocating having a conversation." I didn't really get to his concern about anxiety because I wanted to lock antlers on the technical question, which I thought was a red herring. Some doctors would rather have a fight about science than admit that a conversation makes them uncomfortable.

Jon picked up the thread. "The worry that asking about ACEs creates anxiety and that everybody who has ACEs requires a mental health intervention is something we also hear often. We think it is more common that the person who tells you about ACEs is okay with talking about it – they know what happened, they have it sorted, more or less. They aren't anxious about talking about it – they probably don't want to dwell on it, but they aren't freaked by your question. More importantly, asking doesn't create the problem. That's like saying that asking about suicidality makes someone suicidal. That is very clearly not the way it works. ACE inquiry is like that ... even asking can help, and if it is present, and if for this person it is an unresolved source of distress, then the attention and validation alone can be therapeutic, and you and the person can then set out figuring out next steps. Some of those folks will require more mental health intervention, that's true, but you wouldn't overlook, I don't know, something like alcohol misuse just because the services for it suck, right?"

I was hoping the next question might be less confrontational and was relieved when someone from the back walked forward to ask, "I came to this presentation instead of the other ones in this time slot because I am totally convinced about this stuff. I have been asking my new patients about ACEs for a year or two now. It is easy. You said you're not advocating questionnaires, but I'm wondering if giving everyone a questionnaire might be a good idea."

Jon answered, "Well, we are believers in the idea that you can't tell ahead of time who has ACE and who doesn't. We have been routinely surprised about who confirms ACEs and how intense that experience has been for some folks who look just fine. Like I said, all kinds of people look like they are doing okay ... they don't look like they are carrying a big load. We often hear someone say 'I've never told anyone this before,' and often those folks appreciate the chance to share it, knowing it will be confidential.

"The glitch for me is the questionnaire. Imagine you have never even met a doc, and they ask you for your health card number, address, height, weight, and then ACE history ... and you don't even know if they are the kind of doc you want to work with yet. That could be off-putting, right? So, as clinicians we always see somebody first and ask them in person about ACEs so we can get a sense of how it is affecting them. We might adjust our inquiry based on how they are doing. But it isn't unusual for me to start the inquiry in person, and then invite the person to do a few questionnaires to get a sense of how they stand. If you do it that way, it is a collaborative thing you and the patient are doing together, not a kind of uncontextualized question that can be intrusive and unempathic."

A family doctor that Jon and I both know stood up. It's always reassuring to know the next question is coming from a friend. "I do shifts in the Emergency Department. I was seeing this young guy there last week, from a hostel. He was looking for pain medication. He had a pretty bad skin infection, but he wasn't interested in antibiotics. I couldn't figure out what to do at first, and then I thought, *Oh, yeah, I'll FIFE him.*"

There were nods of appreciation around the room. FIFE is an acronym that family doctors use to remind them to be patient centered when asking about a medical problem. The letters remind them to ask about feelings (e.g., concerns and fears about coping), ideas (personal explanations about what is going on), functioning (how the problem is affecting them), and expectations (what they hope for from the appointment).

Our friend continued, "And that helped establish a conversation, as it usually does, so I could get him to take antibiotics. The point is that FIFE is like second nature to us now and it opens up conversations that help. I'm thinking that maybe asking about ACEs is like that."

Jon replied, "Couldn't agree more. There are a lot of memory aids like that, strategies for getting to important stuff quickly and keeping it in mind. If you already have a strategy, then feel free to just modify it. Our message is not that you have to do this in some perfect way, rather that it is useful to get to it any way that works for you. If you like FIFE, and use it routinely, then maybe just integrate CARE into that."

This discussion was much livelier than is typical after an academic talk. We were the last talk of the day and nobody was leaving, so we just continued. Someone else spoke out from his seat without waiting for a nod. "I'm glad you bring up the Emergency Department. I can see asking new patients in my office about ACEs, but I can't see it in the Emergency Department. Assessment needs to be so focused."

"Sure," Jon agreed. "We aren't trying to get you to do this *every* time you see a patient for *anything* – clinical judgment will always trump rules. But the same ideas apply to the ED as much as they do to a clinic. ACEs make it more likely that someone will be in the ED *and* more likely that they will struggle with dealing with your remedy for their problem. Years ago, we had a woman who came very frequently to our ED for really serious self-harm behavior. She was angry when she came, acting like the staff were her enemies, but still coming day after day for care. It was untenable; staff dreaded seeing her, and even if she let them help, they knew she would be back in a day or two – maybe even later that same day with the same problem. Different services involved, psychiatry or surgery or medicine, would fight with one another, seeing the others as not doing enough. It wasn't until we had a combined meeting with, like, six services, including bioethics, that we figured out a plan that let us all manage her without coming apart at the seams. Once the patients and care providers were having calmer encounters, we were able to ask her about ACEs. Really, to be honest, we were just asking to understand how we could help her instead of repulsing her. Sure enough, she had a terrible childhood – adopted, abused, shamed, abandoned, and in mental health care as a kid from the get-go. She was never experienced as being anything but a problem to the people around her. She expected rejection and denigration from any caregiver and preemptively fought them off, even if she needed their expertise. After we got the plan together, things settled enough that she started coming to psychiatry appointments, and her presentations to the ED tailed right off. That's a dramatic case, for sure, but it does show how getting at the root of this stuff can help. Putting the plan and the ACE awareness in place saved the ED hours and hours of time, and untold expense in terms of procedures, security watches, and so on."

I interjected, "That story may undermine our point about how asking about adversity doesn't usually lead to a need for mental health care. I just want to emphasize that Jon just picked one of the most challenging Emergency Department cases that our hospital has ever managed as an example."

"I'm wondering about trauma-informed care," came a voice from the back. "It looks to me like that could involve overhauling everything we do. I don't see how that is possible in the short run. What can we actually do, other than just asking about ACEs?"

"We could talk about that all day, but since I see we are already past our time, I'll give you a list instead." I counted my instructions off on my fingers as I spoke. "You can start by becoming aware of the role of adversity in your patients' lives. Emphasize your patients' strengths over their pathology. Try to wonder 'what happened to you?' when your reflex response is 'what is wrong with you?' Recognize that managing illness is at least as important a part of the job as treating disease. Listen before you speak; lead with your ears. Believing your patients and validating their experience is therapeutic. Reject the idea that symptoms are either 'real' or psychological; they are almost always both. And, finally, watch out for yourself. Health care is a high-risk occupation. Each of us makes choices that may increase or decrease the risk. Don't treat your own suffering as a weakness or a reason for shame. Take time for yourself. Keep your people near. Speak up when you need to. The one in three statistic applies to us too."

"Maybe one more comment or question?" Jon offered the room.

Someone who hadn't spoken yet stood up. "I'm coming around to this, but I'm not there yet. I can see the evidence. I get that these experiences matter to patients. But my experience is that it is irrelevant for some patients, so why ask? For others the current mental health struggles are so obvious that we are already treating them. I don't see the point of asking those people about old experiences they can't change. We're not doing therapy. And then I guess there is an in-between group for whom it matters but I don't know about it. Maybe if I could recognize who belongs to that group I would ask. I don't know."

"Well, I'm going to be a bit confrontational with you here," Jon responded, with a tone that didn't sound confrontational at all. "I hope that's okay. The reason I'm going in this direction is because I think you've been brave enough to articulate what others in this room are probably thinking but don't want to risk saying out loud. So, I want to thank you for the opportunity to actually confront these very real reactions. But I hope I might be able to convince you that although these reactions are common, they are mostly resistances, feelings that make us shy away from this unhappy topic. They don't actually make medical sense. Here goes!

"Number 1. We ask patients *all* the time about things that don't apply to them. My guess would be that most questions a doctor asks are met with negatives. We do that to create a kind of field in which the positive symptoms really stand out. Pertinent negatives are crucial. So, I'm saying that not asking about something because it may be 'frequently irrelevant' is a departure from what we usually do."

"Number 2. We ask about things that can't change all the time as well. The most obvious example is family history – if someone has multiple cases of cancer in their family because they have a BrCa1 gene, we don't ignore it because we can't change it. We use it to structure care, referrals, prognosis, need for support. Same with ACEs. And if this person is already in oncology care, would you really not care to know it, like you're saying about a person with ACEs already in therapy?

"Your third point, that you don't do therapy, I also think maybe misses the mark. There is a ton of doctor contact that is therapeutic, even if it isn't formally psychotherapy. The presence of a strong alliance where there is trust and agreement about shared goals and strategies is a significant component of what makes psychotherapy – and maybe any treatment – work. That's why we are proselytizing here. The simple appreciation and validation of a person's experience is often highly therapeutic, in fact it is often all the 'therapy' that is needed, to help them affiliate with you in a more trusted therapeutic relationship that can improve their health over the long term – like your colleague did when she decided to ask about bad things in her patient's life.

"Ultimately, you can't identify that perfect group for whom the question is the most relevant unless you ask most people, most of the time. ACEs is not a happy topic, but it is part of your practice whether you ask about it or not. Remember, only 40 per cent of the general population has an ACE score of zero, so we might as well connect with each other about it."

THE CARE METHOD OF ASKING PATIENTS ABOUT CHILDHOOD ADVERSITY

The name of the CARE method can help you remember its four steps: consent, asking, reflection, and engagement.

It starts with getting consent. A simple consent question would be this: "Some childhood and young adult experiences that are pretty common, but difficult, can affect your health later in life. I'd like to ask you about things that may have happened when you were younger. Is that okay?"

Or if you are already talking about a clinical condition that suggests a higher likelihood of ACEs, like chronic pain, addiction, or depression, you could use that for context. Let's say you are talking with someone about recurrent headaches. You could say: "Since we're talking about chronic pain, I'd like to ask about some childhood and young adult experiences that are common in this situation. Is that okay?"

If the patient indicates that it is okay to go on, then the next step is A, for asking. When asking about ACEs, you don't have to be precise. It may be better to give a little list that conveys the general idea. The list sort of gives your patient permission to describe other similar things.

You might say: "When you were young, did you have experiences that were frightening or that made you feel unsafe? For example, were you hit, or touched in a way that you didn't want, or bullied? Did you feel unprotected or unloved?"

The most important part of asking is actually listening to how your patient responds. If they start telling you something in the middle of your question, stop and listen. If they tell you they don't want to talk about it, acknowledge that and move on. Listening well and following your patient's cues are the most important parts.

So that's C, consent, and A, asking. If your patient doesn't want to talk about it, or doesn't have anything to report, then you're done, and it's probably taken less than a minute.

If they have something to tell you, move on to R for reflecting and E for engaging.

To reflect on what has been said, you validate what your patient has told you and indicate that you're willing to think and talk about it together.

You can say: "Thank you for sharing that. Sometimes experiences like that have an impact on how you respond to stress later in life. I wonder if you draw any connection between those events and your current situation." Again, it's vital to listen to how your patient responds.

The final step is to engage. In this step you defer to your patient about what comes next.

You can say: "Are you comfortable sharing more with me?" or "Is this something you would like to talk more about at another time?"

Listen to what your patient says and follow their lead. Many people are content to have shared something relevant and don't need to talk more.

And that's it. You're done.

Working to help doctors who are set in their ways to pay attention to childhood adversity is worthwhile, and we put a lot of effort into it, but it is a pre-revolutionary activity. It isn't going to change the world. A better way to make changes is to train young doctors differently.

Health Care Students

Sometimes I get a chance to teach medical students during the first week of their first year. Leading a group discussion of students right at the start of medical school might be a cure for burnout in old, tired, veteran doctors. The students are smart and enthusiastic. Most don't have much medical knowledge, and they have few skills, but they often know a lot about the social determinants of health, and they are full of compassion.

During their medical training, most of them will become *less* empathic. We select students who are perfectly suited to practice patient-centered, empathic, holistic care and then we squeeze it out of them over several years of medical training. We turn those better souls into us – impatient partialists, dismissive of soft skills like listening well.

Those years of training also threaten the students' mental health – the two processes go hand in hand. An alarming number of them will be showing signs of professional burnout before they have even acquired a license to treat patients. Some will even die by suicide. Unhealthy and unreasonable expectations for how much a person can work and a system that demands responsibility but provides insufficient support contribute. Perhaps most malignantly, we model a culture in which reflection, self-compassion, and compassion for one another are exceptional. How can we teach our students to cure sometimes, relieve often, comfort always when we don't even treat ourselves and one another that way?

So, medical culture must change. But beyond that, we also need to teach future health care professionals how to act and why. They will be exposed to real-world patients from very early in their training and much of the teaching is framed in clinical scenarios known as case-based learning. Communication skills will be emphasized, and students benefit from experiential learning, such as by receiving immediate and detailed feedback from observed practice interviews with actors who are trained to play the role of patients. Currently, incorporation of the role of childhood trauma and other forms of adversity is usually modest, perhaps being written into some of the clinical scenarios that are used as the basis for discussion in case-based learning. At some medical schools, cases have been developed expressly to introduce trauma-informed care, but that is exceptional. These excellent exceptions are one-off experiences, like workshops. Fighting for space in the medical school curriculum can be intense, so these are victories. Nonetheless, teaching that actually shapes behavior is much more intense than what can be provided in a workshop: it is repeated, experiential, observed, and coached.

If we are going to change how new generations of doctors think about childhood adversity, they also need knowledge. In the same way that students learn about risk factors for cardiac disease or diabetes through repeated encounters with the information in classroom learning, in formal and informal discussions, in their bedside teaching, and on their exams, the relevance of trauma needs to be embedded in their learning in all subjects. We have a great deal to review, discuss, and apply, from the scientific statement of the American Heart Association that "substantial evidence documents an association between childhood adversity and cardiometabolic outcomes across the life course" to evidence of the importance of ACEs to cancer, lung disease, infectious disease, and the rest. After repeatedly hearing that ACEs matter to whatever specialty of medicine in which they are training, students will incorporate it in their thinking about their clinical work automatically, like they do genetics and exposures to cigarettes and alcohol. For the next generation of students, ACEs would be part of ordinary medicine, not a special topic.

Knowledge only gets you so far. Altering the content of the medical curriculum doesn't change what doctors *do*. The more formative change occurs when we address *process*, how health care professionals use their knowledge, how they act and interact. We need to support our new doctors' abilities to demonstrate empathy. We need to prepare them for the discomfort they will feel with patients who distrust them or who refuse to follow good advice or send desperate messages of need. They need to practice difficult interactions, which is best accomplished through encounters with simulated patients who are observed and coached. These simulations allow them to take a chance, risk failing or harming a "patient" without any dire consequences, and learn from their experience. Typically, in such simulations students observe each other in groups, vicariously learning from others' experience.

New doctors need to appreciate the experience of people who have grown up with substantial adversity, even if they themselves have not. Isaac could teach them a thing or two – teaching designed in collaboration with those who have the personal experience that is being taught can be much more effective.

Perhaps students could assess their own ACE scores privately as they learn about the relevance of these experiences for their patients, as a tool to enrich discussion. Instruction in how to ask about trauma in general, and childhood trauma in particular, could be embedded in the parts of the curriculum in which they learn interviewing skills and practice FIFE, to learn about their patient's feelings, ideas, function, and expectations.

The hidden curriculum of medical culture, which emphasizes the distinction between "us and them" and is more comfortable with biology and disease than with relationship and illness, is a powerful foe to the kinds of change in medical education we are advocating. That is why change may take an educational generation or two. It may take that long to have teachers who believe in the curriculum.

One way to accelerate change is to link the revolution in trauma-informed care to complementary disruptive forces from anti-racist, feminist, and queer perspectives, which all aim to overturn oppressive elements of the health care culture. The Care Revolution must stand shoulder to shoulder with these critiques of the status quo on health care. An extra workshop or two is not going to get us where we need to go.

Health and Child Welfare Organizations

Alan is a cop from a town near Glasgow in Scotland. He was on the same walking tour of Prague beerhouses with Lynn and me in the autumn of 2018, and we shared a table for an hour or two at the last pub on the tour. I was more talkative than usual after sampling the local fare; Alan is probably always like that. I was wearing a T-shirt from the tour of a band I like that Alan hadn't heard of, which got us talking about music. The conversation became enthusiastic when we realized we shared more than our taste in bands and beer. Alan was vocal about his pride in the fact that his entire police force is ACE aware. In fact, much of Scotland is. The walking tour was just a few weeks after a conference held by ACE-Aware Scotland, whose vision is "to ensure that an entire nation ... every single citizen of Scotland understand[s] the impact of childhood distress." Alan recounted police calls to respond to situations of drunkenness or family violence and his new perspective on trying to understand who was at risk and how to help. Alan's testimony suggests Scotland is far ahead of most nations. We have a long way to go before most public-facing services are attuned to trauma.

Within the health care system, the revolution that awaits is trauma-informed care, as I described in Chapter 19. Its principles emphasize sharing power in health care, training nonclinical and clinical staff members to be aware of trauma, collaborating, maintaining safety, focusing on strengths rather than deficits and on recovery rather than treatment, and avoiding secondary trauma. There has been more progress adopting trauma-informed care in the child welfare sector than in health care organizations. However, even in that sector, most organizations have not reached the goal.

To get a sense of the challenges, I talked to Dr. Wendy Manel, a psychologist at the Catholic Children's Aid Society in Ontario, who has championed trauma-informed care there for over five years: "Over time, we have tried to shift our practice, but when the entire roots of the system are focused on intervening with how people behave, rather than on understanding why this is happening and promoting recovery and support, it is hard to change."

She explained that child welfare organizations were first formed in North America in the late nineteenth century to provide social services to homeless "street urchins" and impoverished families, who were often immigrants, in cities such as New York and Toronto. The motto of the Toronto Children's Aid Society, founded in 1891, was "It is wiser and less expensive to save children then to punish criminals." Laws were enacted to permit these organizations to apprehend children from the street or from neglectful families, often placing them in industrial schools. The focus was on discipline and the risk of criminality. "It was not trauma informed at all," Dr. Manel said. "No one was asking, 'What happened to you?' It was all about 'What is wrong with you?' and trying to get kids in line. The foundation of child welfare was for the state to assess what is wrong with a family and intervene to correct a problem."

"So, it was about blame and apprehension from the start?"

"Not always apprehension. But yes, it was very problem focused. The sector as a whole has been very crisis driven and reactive. Shifts in our approach tend to happen after something really bad happens. Our policies are shaped by high-profile child deaths – which are fortunately rare – through a risk-averse and problem-focused lens, so it is hard to shift.

"Before we started to make the shift toward trauma-informed care at our agency, there was an effort to implement a program that paid attention to attachment, and loss, and trauma, but it was all focused on just the kids. I said, 'You are fixing one tire on a car that is headed down a hill very quickly. If you are trying to help a kid in a foster home that doesn't know how to support them, and they are not receiving services that complement that, that car is still going downhill.'"

I asked if the organization resisted the idea of shifting toward trauma-informed care.

"No, they were right on board. Although some of our leaders were surprised that we were conceptualizing trauma in this broader sense that includes chronic neglect and other things, not just physical and sexual abuse ... One of the things that happens in child welfare is you get exposed to so much that you lose perspective. I like the concept of *toxic stress*, which includes a broad range of experiences that are bad for brain development. But some of these things feel 'like nothing' after doing this work for a while. But getting the organization on side was the easy part. Change is slow."

"Can you give me an example of what is changing?"

"We are much less intrusive now at the point of first contact with families. We are much more likely to be linking them with resources in their own communities. I would credit this to efforts for us to adopt anti-racist and anti-oppressive practice, which is very complementary to trauma-informed care and comes from the recognition that there is an over-representation of Black and Indigenous children in care. Or, for another example, we do a lot of advocacy with schools now so that we are working together to help families and kids who are struggling. We used to just be brought in as the heavy when there was a lot of truancy and they couldn't get a kid into school."

"What are the biggest barriers?"

"You can't change one system without changes in the other systems we work with. We work with the justice system and the health care system, for example. We can't refer a family to resources that don't exist or that have a two-year wait-list.

"For a concrete example, we were working with a foster family that knew they were having trouble raising foster kids because of their own past experiences with trauma and loss. So, the obvious next step would be to get some therapy for the foster parents, but our funding model doesn't allow for that. We can get resources for the kids but not for the foster parents.

"Also, there are so many other changes that our workers are trying to manage at the same time. We have been shifting from paper notes to a computerized system and a shared database with other child welfare organizations, which are really important, useful changes, but our workers can only manage so much change at the same time.

"One of the things we want to do that we haven't yet is to develop comprehensive training for our foster parents on how to parent children who have been exposed to toxic stress." (See the "Parents" section, below, for examples of how to do that.)

Dr. Manel spoke of the "parallel process," the ways in which child welfare workers are treated and react in ways that are similar to the clients they are serving. "I think the work is very hard on them. They are great. But we send them into situations where they need to be concerned about their own safety and where they are exposed to others' trauma. In child welfare, we adapt just like everyone else who is exposed to trauma adapts. We become trauma averse and reactive, and we focus on the immediate risk, not the long-term risk to kids. The majority of our cases are not about physical abuse or sexual abuse; they are about chronic issues like domestic violence, neglect, mental health and addictions, and the consequences of racism and poverty. Our workers don't get training in how to manage the very emotionally heavy part of their work. Until recently, we haven't really focused on the secondary trauma our people experience.

"I'm trying to bring a trauma-informed perspective to everything we do. And other child welfare organizations are trying to make these changes, but everyone is 'choosing their own adventure.' There isn't a standard way to do this ... But it feels urgent to me. Every day we are not practicing trauma-informed care is a day we are not serving our children as well as we could."

Although the challenges to adopting trauma-informed care are large for child welfare organizations, they will be much greater for health care organizations, where we can't assume that leaders will be "right on board" at the start. A more attainable goal may be trauma awareness, such as has been adopted by Alan's police force. The goal for that baby step is for all members of the organization to learn of the impact of trauma and appreciate the role it plays in their clients' lives.

Parents

A Care Revolution that aims for prevention and early intervention needs to provide resources that allow parents to be their best selves. There is good evidence that a stepped approach to attachment-based teaching and support for new parents could greatly improve the lives of children: some teaching for all, more intensive training for those who want it, professional relation-based support for those at greater risk, and intensive behavioral coaching for those whose needs are greatest.

Three parenting resources that draw on attachment theory to help parents to raise safe and secure children provide a good example of the possibilities for a step-wise approach to parenting supports. Although these examples are independent interventions that are not organized in a stepped-care approach currently, they could be. In such an approach, the least intensive and most accessible resources would be available to all while the most intensive and expensive resources are saved for those with the greatest needs.

The Circle of Security program provides resources that are accessible to all parents. The program is based on much evidence that parental responsiveness to a child's emotional states is a key to obtaining security. Being responsive involves skills like reading a child's cues and being able to take the time to reflect on the child's mental state so one can remain attentive and responsive in spite of the pull of one's own emotional reactions. The Circle of Security program provides educational resources and more intensive training programs. Research on the more intensive form of training showed that a significant portion of children who have an insecure attachment when their parents start the training have a secure attachment afterward.

The Nurse-Family Partnership in the United States involves home visits by nurses for low-income, first-time mothers. It aims to improve the health of babies at birth, improve child health and development, including reducing child maltreatment, and improve mothers' lives in the long run by helping them, for example, to return to school and find work. Nurses visit about weekly and help women by encouraging them to set small, achievable goals and to use problem-solving skills, with the intent that accomplishing goals will enhance their sense of self-efficacy when facing further challenges. Nurses emphasize the mother's strengths and endeavor to get other family members and friends involved in the pregnancy, birth, and care of the baby. They act as navigators to help the mother and her family members connect to other support services as needed. The *relationship* between the nurse, the mother, and her family is the foundation of this work.

Robust scientific evaluation has shown that the Nurse-Family Partnership improves the lives of mothers and their children for many years. In the early years, child abuse and neglect were reduced by 48 per cent and emergency room visits for accidents and poisoning by 56 per cent. Women in the treatment group had a longer period between their first and second babies and more stable partnerships, and their kids did better in school. By the time the kids were nine, it was possible to detect lower child mortality rates. After eighteen years, benefits continued to accrue. The net cost was negative. The program saves money.

The most intensive early parenting intervention in this series of steps is the Attachment Biobehavioral Catch-Up (ABC) program, which was developed by Dr. Mary Dozier at the University of Delaware. It is intended for young children and toddlers who have experienced substantial adversity, such as those in foster care, having come from homes with poverty, substance abuse, mental illness, physical illness, or violence. Most have experienced some form of abuse or neglect.

ABC targets the emotional, behavioral, and biological dysregulation these kids experience. ABC coaches work intensively with foster parents or birth parents, providing very specific support and instruction: teaching caregivers to follow the child's lead; helping caregivers to appreciate the value of touching, cuddling, and hugging their child; and helping caregivers create conditions that allow their children to express emotions and to learn to recognize and understand emotions. Each of these goals aims to change behaviors rather than attitudes. It is an intense but brief intervention – just ten sessions. ABC reduces by almost half the most severe types of attachment dysregulation in these high-risk kids.

Circle of Security, Nurse-Family Partnership, and ABC could form a stepped approach to improving care within families: something for everyone, according to need.

Citizens

Some aspects of the Care Revolution require new directions in public policy – and so they depend on the voices and votes of citizens. This certainly applies to changes that will prevent more kids from suffering Isaac's fate. It also applies to changes that are urgently needed to help those who are living with the consequences of childhood maltreatment to recover.

Compared to other survivors of childhood traumas, Isaac's situation is atypical in one important way – he has been seeing a psychiatrist for psychotherapy for twenty years. That is just not available to most people. In fact, there is compelling evidence that psychiatrists who see the same patients for many years, as I have done with Isaac, create a barrier to others receiving needed psychiatric care – essentially, all the people I didn't see using more time-limited interventions during the hours I have spent with Isaac.

High-quality psychotherapy is an effective treatment for many mental illnesses, including most of those caused by childhood adversity. So, one thing that needs to change in health care for the system to meet the mental health needs of those who were exposed to severe adversity as children is increased access to high-quality psychotherapy. It is a long-standing problem.

In 2012, a lack of counseling was the most frequent unmet need of Canadians with mental health challenges, and access was worse for those with lower incomes. Canada's universal health care system covers psychotherapy delivered by physicians at no direct cost to those receiving it; it does not pay for the same therapy delivered by a psychologist or other qualified psychotherapist, who must be paid out of pocket or by an insurer. Inequities are essentially built into the system.

In the United States, the economics of health care are very different, but problems with access to mental health care are similar. Almost ninety million Americans live in regions that the federal government has designated as having a shortage of mental health professionals. Of those with unmet needs for mental health care, 45 per cent cite cost as a barrier. It is worse for Mexican Americans, Black people, and presumably other racialized people.

The United Kingdom has demonstrated a way forward by putting a massive effort into implementing a model called Increased Access to Psychotherapy, which has provided service to millions of citizens in its first few years. It provides stepped care, meaning that people with more severe illness get more intense treatment from therapists with more expertise. The first step is advice from people who have some training, which might include direction to self-help resources. If a person has more severe anxiety or depression, or has post-traumatic stress disorder, they are referred to an evidence-based therapy, like cognitive-behavioral therapy. The most specialized and intense services are reserved for those who need them. Some have a single session; most continue. The results are promising, in terms of both the benefits that people receive and the ability to provide more care at a sustainable cost.

A PARTNER'S PERSPECTIVE ON GETTING CARE FOR THE CONSEQUENCES OF TRAUMA

Heather Tuba's husband, Derek, lives with the consequences of trauma. He has complex symptoms that include dissociation ("spacing out" or becoming disconnected from one's surroundings for a time), which can happen when a person who has experienced trauma is caught up in re-experiencing old events and loses track of their actual surroundings. It can be very frightening or bewildering. Heather has gained so much experience supporting Derek as his partner that she now provides resources and education to other partners in her position.

"Having navigated both the public medical and mental health system and the private psychotherapy system ... I have experienced the big gaps in what is available for people with complex trauma. Medical practitioners, including many psychiatrists, don't understand complex trauma. We have a really good family doctor, but his understanding of the medications that can help is very limited. Wait times for treatment are many months long, and then the treatments are short – a few weeks. Communication between practitioners is poor; it is not clear whose fault it is when planned follow-up fails, as it has done.

"Trauma work relies heavily on the capacity to feel safe, but Derek has received suggestions that felt quite unsafe from specialists who are new to him and not planning to continue to see him. That has dysregulated his emotions ... He has been treated in hospital, but short stays with no supports in place at the time of discharge are not helpful to someone who needs to feel safe. We found outpatient treatment that was offered in the public system was not a good match; treatments were offered that can make dissociation worse.

"We have had a better experience with a private psychotherapist, but it was not easy to find the right one. It took four tries to find someone who had the specific skills and training to deal with his dissociation. It goes beyond being trauma informed ... The therapy that is working is long-term therapy, based on models developed by trauma experts.

"I think what helped us to persist and find the right therapy was that we have an excellent private insurance plan, so we could afford to keep trying; I have contacts through my online work that enabled me to get the right name; Derek and I are educated, so we can read and search for resources. We have quite a few advantages – it shouldn't be necessary to have all of that to get good care."

We asked Heather what the system requires. She had a thoughtful list:

- We need access to psychotherapists who have the specific skills to work with complex trauma, specifically dissociation, specific guidelines about what that encompasses, and a database of clinicians who have training to work with this population.
- There is a public responsibility to prevent childhood adversity, but equally, there is a responsibility to repair damage and injury to adults who were once vulnerable children.
- The system needs education programs about childhood trauma to better understand the impact of neglect, attachment trauma, witnessing interpersonal violence and aggression, and verbal abuse. This can also include racism, immigration trauma, gun violence, and so on.
- Recognition of childhood trauma as a determinant of physical, mental, social health, and longevity. For example, Derek has issues with chronic pain, but no one has asked about history beyond the physical health or accidents.
- There is a need for greater recognition of how common dissociation is for people who have experienced trauma, including people who develop addictions.

Heather also told us about the personal challenges: "Treatment is expensive. That affects the whole family. Finding treatment also has a mental and an emotional cost. I've become somewhat of a specialist by need. I often know more than the medical staff and sometimes the therapist, but professionals dismiss my judgment. Partners are also left out of the process because of confidentiality.

"Derek and I always want our relationship to work but having no one to explain how trauma works and how it disrupts many day-to-day functions makes it very challenging. It has affected employment for both of us. It has placed incredible stress on our relationship and our children. Marriage counseling is often inadequate because the therapists have such limited knowledge of trauma. My mental and physical health have suffered. This definitely affects my sleep and overall stress levels, and my physical health.

"I have very little social support. I have worked very hard to build a support network for myself and I have learned to be quite choosy about who that is! This topic is a conversation stopper for many people."

Since Heather now provides support and resources to others' partners, we asked what common themes she observes. "Partners struggle with exhaustion, fear of the future, worry about parenting, a desire to maintain the relationship but also to draw some boundaries. The symptoms, such as intense emotions changing suddenly with no apparent trigger, can be very confusing to people who don't understand trauma and don't know how the brain works. Many are too worn out to do much reading, although they try because the burden of education falls on the family. In some ways, there is too much information out there about trauma and in other ways, not enough.

"Many partners are told to find a therapist for themselves but are disappointed that therapists don't understand complex trauma. Partners need to be able to manage their own overwhelmed nervous systems. Many partners are not looking for their own therapy; they want normalization and tools to manage. Many relationships do not last because people are worn out and confused by the symptoms.

"With increasing awareness of trauma and access to information via the internet, couples may recognize the signs that one or both experienced childhood trauma. The sooner they can access support, the greater the opportunity to lessen the impact over their lifespan, including the effect on interpersonal relationships.

Early intervention in adulthood can prevent the reinforcement of physiological and psychological trauma responses that are prevalent with unaddressed trauma. I know if Derek had received the support he needed in his twenties, he may not have experienced some of the fallout in his life. As a family, we certainly would not have gone through as much confusion and stress."

Preventing childhood maltreatment is the most revolutionary idea. It is possible but can't happen without a revolution in public values, because currently no society can claim that its citizens hold a shared belief that harming children is wrong, that it is not justified by the autonomy of parents or by a balance of benefits and harms, and that it is worth the cost of eliminating it.

The policy strategies that have been recommended to prevent ACEs are far-reaching: change social norms to support parents and positive parenting; enhance parenting skills to promote healthy child development; strengthen economic supports to families; improve other social determinants of health, including gender inequality, discrimination based on race, ethnicity, LGBTQ2+ identity, or disability, barriers to education, problematic substance use, and poverty and homelessness; and provide quality care and education early in life. Some add the strategy of punishing abusers and supporting victims, although the impact of those strategies on the greater goal of prevention is questionable.

Examples of policy goals and initiatives to match these strategies and approaches could compose the platform of the most unelectable political party imaginable: universal minimum income, child-tax benefits, health and disability insurance, unemployment insurance, parental postnatal leave, affordable high-quality day care, harm-reduction strategies and decriminalization of drugs, community mental health crisis services by mental health experts rather than police, affordable postsecondary school tuition, affordable housing initiatives, public education campaigns, legislation to outlaw corporal punishment, enhanced parental support programs, enhanced mental health support, early detection and intervention for children experiencing abuse including in schools, and enhanced child and youth mental health and addiction services.

As a block, these initiatives are enormously expensive. This is an opportune point to recall that the estimated cost of child abuse, just for those cases reported and verified during childhood (a vast underestimate) and just in the United States, is $2 trillion. So, the costs of expensive initiatives are likely to be more than offset by their benefits. But arguments like that are often unpersuasive when the repayment is many election cycles after the investment.

There have been successes in this direction already, but they are incremental, not revolutionary. Take systemic racism directed toward Indigenous children in Canada as an example. In 2015, Canada's Truth and Reconciliation Commission made ninety-four specific calls for action in many domains that include reducing the disproportionate number of Indigenous children in provincial and territorial care and Indigenous adults in prison, eliminating barriers to education, creating legislation to preserve Indigenous languages, acknowledging that the state of Indigenous health in Canada is a direct result of previous Canadian government policies, and overcoming jurisdictional and funding barriers to health care. By 2019, just nine of the ninety-four calls had been implemented.

Changes in criminal law could contribute to culture shift. The so-called spanking law provides an example. Dr. Tracie Afifi (whose study of abuse histories among soldiers we described in Chapter 2) cites twenty years of research that demonstrates "that spanking is associated with an increased probability of mental health problems, substance use, suicidal ideation/attempts, and physical health conditions along with developmental, behavioral, social, and cognitive problems. Importantly, there are no studies indicating that hitting a child as a means of discipline is beneficial for the child." Yet in Canada, physical violence that would otherwise be considered assault under the Criminal Code is legal if the person receiving the force is a child and the one using the force is the child's teacher, parent, or a person standing in place of a parent (like a babysitter), provided that the force used is reasonable and that it is used for the purpose of correction. The latter caveat presupposes that using force ever serves as an effective corrective for children, which is dubious.

The spanking issue remains contentious, although the tide is shifting in children's favor. Corporal punishment in schools is illegal in most European countries and about half of American states, although it is legal in Canada. While the majority of Americans favor allowing parents to decide about physical discipline, about half of European countries have outlawed corporal punishment at home. In 2016, 57 per cent of Canadians regarded spanking a child as "always or usually morally wrong."

Repeal of the spanking exception to assault laws would not have a large public health impact in itself. Countries that have banned corporal punishment do not always witness a change in parents' behavior. But it is an example of a concrete legislative step whose intent is to change values and attitudes. Shifting the conversation about corporal punishment from one about parents' right to choose to one of children's human rights, from autonomy to public health, is the goal.

Since there are so many expert consensus road maps and guides on to how to reduce child maltreatment, one has to assume that the government bodies and organizations that sponsor them recognize the need, at some level. So why are kids today as likely to grow up with Isaac's experiences as he was? It is hard not to conclude that the fundamental problem is a lack of political will to maintain these challenges as priorities. Which raises the question of how to change political will. Perhaps implementing the policy changes that have been proposed to prevent child maltreatment will require electoral reform. In Canada, two reforms that have been suggested are eliminating first-past-the-post elections in favor of some form of proportional representation and lowering the voting age to sixteen. In the United States, where changes might need to occur state by state, the challenges are different. Each nation will have its own solutions.

Patients

What do we do until the revolution comes? Many people seem to start from the reflex response that if you suffered some kind of important exposure to adversity as a kid, then you need mental health treatment. That is just not true. Here are some other ideas to reflect on to get the best health care available.

Make as honest and compassionate an inventory as you can about what happened, how it affects you, and your strengths and vulnerabilities. As we have argued before, it isn't your ACE score that matters nearly as much as a clear vision of how you have responded to the things that happened as a kid that lead to feeling unsafe, uncared for, or less than worthy. Still, calculating your ACE score may have some value, if only to see where you fit with respect to everyone else. We have talked to many people who tend to minimize the impact of their childhood exposure and frame it all as normal, but who have been taken aback to see that with an ACE score of four, for example, they are in the top 15 per cent of adverse exposure and in a high-risk category with respect to physical and mental health problems in the future. There is a link to an online ACE calculator using the original ten categories in the endnotes if you are curious.

Think about how you have responded to adversity. Be as honest as you can, and also be generous to yourself. Adapting is a strength. Developing defenses is exactly what you would hope to do when under siege. Still, the responses that were the best defense against threats and harm long ago may not be serving you well now. That's how it works for everyone – we overreact to threats that don't materialize, we protect ourselves at the cost of getting less out of our lives, we miscalculate blame toward ourselves and others. Try to keep an open mind about things you have heard about yourself repeatedly – maybe there is a grain of truth there, even if it hurt to hear at the time.

Everyone is different – different exposure, different response, and different context. So generic advice should raise suspicions. All the more so because adverse experiences seem to push some people in one direction and others in the opposite direction with respect to some important responses and consequences. It puts us in the position of the dermatologist in an old medical joke who advises, "If it's wet, keep it dry; if it's dry, keep it wet." Rather than giving generic advice, for some challenges we will do what we think is more useful: we will frame guidance in terms of common tensions between opposite poles so that you can locate yourself on each continuum.

Oversharing versus withholding. Some people feel so unsafe and unable to manage independently that they can't contain anxieties, worries, hurts, and resentments; they need to express them. If you are like this, your oversharing may make it hard for those around you to help because your suffering may feel indiscriminant to them. You may wear out your welcome, even with those who really do care about you. It helps to learn to keep some of it to yourself. As with many of the challenges that follow from childhood adversity, there is no quick fix, but it is possible to gain more comfort tolerating your *meshugas*. Mindfulness meditation works for some people to gain an "oh, there I go again" acceptance of perpetual internal turmoil. Cognitive therapy is the formal therapeutic approach to teaching yourself that the things you are fearing are less imminent or likely than you think. There are self-help workbooks and online resources to learn those skills.

On the other hand, if your response to early experiences convinced you that others are so untrustworthy, harmful, or unreliable that your best bet is to keep everything to yourself, you have a different challenge. For one thing, others probably don't know when you need support or help. For another, they probably guess wrong about you fairly often. It is pretty common for reticence to be misinterpreted as arrogance or caginess. It is helpful to take advantage of little opportunities to act against type when they arise – when you are with people who are more reliable listeners or when you recognize a moment that lends itself to greater sharing. Speaking up in those moments can expand your circle of comfort. Be prepared for it to go poorly some of the time – new skills don't arrive fully formed. It can also help to play with nonverbal modes of communicating, like keeping a journal or painting, to experiment with revealing your thoughts and feelings while maintaining a degree of personal control. Isaac found that paying attention to dreams provided a helpful window into his inner world.

Excessive versus insufficient help seeking. Those who overshare are often the same people who frequently ask for support or assistance, sometimes so frequently that it becomes an impediment. In a health care setting, frequent "crises" that turn out to be yet another eruption of virtually constant anxiety can lead to failures of a timely response after a while.

People who are too self-reliant have a different problem. In a health care setting, they will miss opportunities for early intervention because they are not inclined to show up unless things have progressed to an intolerable state. Just as for the avoidant men who don't screen for prostate cancer and women who don't get mammograms or Pap smears, discussed in Chapter 17, reticence to seek help has consequences. In both cases, for those who seek help too much and too little, the sensible solution is the same – meeting with a health care provider, typically a family doctor, regularly rather than as needed. For those whose instinct to seek help has too low a bar, regular appointments provide predictability and a comforting rhythm, and weaken the contingency between asking for help and getting it, which can reduce how urgent it feels to signal need. For those who are reluctant to seek help, the value of meeting a doctor according to a schedule is obvious. It just makes sense to let someone else in on decisions about what you need.

Consider sharing your story. As we have said before, most doctors and other health care professionals of other disciplines are not very good at discussing trauma. Chances are you aren't going to be asked about your childhood adversity. So, it may not feel safe to bring it up; it may feel like the conversation won't be welcome. Fair enough; feeling safe has to come first. But if the conditions feel right, and especially if you are asked, consider being open about your experience. It is relevant and the conversation may help you and the health care providers who know to arrange your health care so that it works better for you.

Manage traumatic memories and avoid re-traumatization. Many medical procedures and treatments are intrusive, some are painful, questions are personal and sometimes catch you by surprise, privacy may be lacking. For many people, what happens in a medical exam or test is close enough to what happened during traumatic events to trigger memories. It needn't be as dramatic as the allergic reaction that made Isaac feel like he was drowning. Often, the connections between current events and memories are subtle and only apparent to the patient – a smell, the tone in someone's voice. Sometimes what happens isn't exactly "remembering"; it is more like having emotional reactions that make more sense in the original situation than the current one.

There may not be much that you can do about reminders that catch you by surprise, but some can be anticipated and avoided or managed. Bringing a confidante to accompany you can make a difference. They should be a silent partner for the most part – the doctor is going to want to talk to you, not to your friend or your sibling – but their presence can be reassuring (and they also serve the purpose of being a second pair of ears in case anxiety interferes with hearing and remembering what you are told). Under the right circumstances, letting the professional who is involved know that the procedure is frightening for you can allow for a collaborative approach. This can work very well, for example, with dental procedures, provided your dentist has the right skills. Note that these two examples of managing around traumatic memories involve including others in the solution. Trying to tough it out by yourself is often part of the problem.

Reject the false dichotomy of physical (real, valid) versus psychological (in your head, imaginary). The conversation between a patient and health care provider about a symptom that doesn't have an obvious explanation or that isn't getting better with the usual treatment is often fraught. Both are likely to fall prey to the trap of the false dichotomy that symptoms are either real or psychological. As we discussed when peeling back six layers of complexity to understand Isaac's pain in Chapter 6, bodily sensations don't work that way. Philosophers may feel that they grew bored of the "mind-body problem" and moved on to other challenges long ago, but actual people whose bodies create trouble and those who try to care for them are still very much stuck on Descartes's division between the material world and the mind. This is such a problem on both sides of the conversation that we give this same advice to health care providers.

On the patients' side of the conversation, rejecting the dichotomy means keeping an open mind to the possibility that physical symptoms are amplified, maintained, and altered by emotions, thoughts, attention, and learning, as well as by mental health conditions like depression and anxiety disorders and, in a generic way, by stress. That doesn't make the symptoms less real. It doesn't even say anything about what caused the symptoms in the first place, just that the forces that affect how they are experienced are many and interact in complicated ways.

Mental illness, post-traumatic stress disorder, and complex PTSD. In spite of being psychiatrists, we have not emphasized mental illness or psychiatric treatments in this book. That is intentional. Although childhood adversity substantially increases the risk of adult mental illnesses, especially depression, anxiety disorders, and substance use disorders, we are trying to change a common and misleading assumption that this is the main problem. We are arguing *against* the idea that everyone who experienced abuse has a mental illness and that medical attention to that trouble should lie mostly in the realm of psychiatry.

Nonetheless, mental illnesses are common and often the most treatable part of a complex mix of medical problems. Specific disorders benefit from specific treatments. Usually, a frank discussion with a family doctor about the symptoms that are interfering with your life is the place to start evaluating what is going on and how to address it.

GETTING THE BEST CARE that is available within the current system is a huge challenge for patients and their families. Jon and I have spent our careers trying to provide the best care that we can within our expertise and to educate and advocate for better care throughout the health care system. One of the reasons this work is so hard is that it starts decades too late for those who have been affected by maltreatment as children, like Isaac.

The work we do is intensive, frustrating, occasionally transformative, but usually cobbled together by patients trying desperately to coordinate their disconnected partialists. The health care system could do better. We could be more trauma informed; we could teach our new professionals what to expect and what to do about it. We could make sure that people like Isaac have access to the therapy they need. But surely the best answer is to come together as a society to prevent harm.

Prevention depends on advocacy, leadership, persistence, and vision. The things that need to change to revolutionize how we support parents and children are mostly known, but they are waiting for advocates, leaders, and visionaries. They are waiting for voters and for the voices of those who are willing to stand in their communities to demand that we raise strong children instead of trying to fix broken adults.

They are waiting for you.

Postscript

Although I usually wait for Isaac to start our session, this time I begin. "We are about to receive a contract to write the book. I don't want to frame this as a question because I've asked so many times that I think it would be irritating ... but now is the time to tell me not to do this. You can still do that."

"Sign the contract. Write the book. Do it."

I paused and Isaac spoke again.

"I had a dream this week. There was a video screen. It was far in the distance so it was really small and hard to see. I was trying to see but it wasn't clear. There were naked people fighting with each other ... Then you came up behind me and you had a remote control. You changed the channel."

Telling Isaac's story is hard. Jon and I expect that reading it is, too. As psychiatrists exposed to many stories like Isaac's, we have often found our motivation to keep going in our anger. Isaac's experiences piss us off because they are so common and yet invisible. They have damaged him for his entire life and yet were entirely preventable. It helps that his long treatment, which has not yet led to healing, has led to hope.

There are millions of adults who live with the consequences of harmful childhood experiences. In that sense, Isaac's story is nothing special; that is the point of telling it. But, of course, it *is* special.

"I've always asked you for everything you have, no half measures," Isaac wrote to Bob at the start of this story. We need to ask of ourselves – every one of us in our privileged and highly resourced society – for the same commitment, no half measures.

Trauma-informed care, healing, and prevention require that we open our eyes to what is right before us and that we tell the truth about it. We don't need any more evidence about how these experiences affect well-being throughout life.

We need change.

Let's summon the courage and humility to accept that we are all a little bit broken and recognize the power that emerges between people who work to respect, understand, and care for each other.

Let's be pissed off together and get this done.

Acknowledgments

Teaching is like a venereal disease. When we teach, our students are taught by everyone who ever taught us. Some of the teachers we had in mind while writing this book are Carol George, Jeremy Holmes, Bill Lancee, Christine Lay, Molyn Leszcz, Patrick Luyten, Clare Pain, Paula Ravitz, Rodney Slonim, Graeme Taylor, and Malcolm West.

We are grateful for those who offered criticism, suggestions, assistance, support, and encouragement, including Amy Bombay, Patricia Cavanagh, Lynn Fisher, David Fisman, Sylvia Fraser, David Goldbloom, Natalie Heeney, Michael Levine, Karen Le, Yona Lunsky, Nancy Mackenzie, Wendy Manel, Katie Maunder, Howard Ovens, Sue Robins, Kathy Soden, Sally Szuster, Heather and Derek Tuba, Ross Upshur, and Lesley Wiesenfeld. Thank you to University of Toronto Press editor Natalie Fingerhut, who offered both enthusiastic support and wise critique, as well as to UTP's whole team, including Lisa Jemison, Anna Del Col, and Chris Reed. We were fortunate, once again, to have our writing improved by Dawn Hunter.

We have been supported in this work by the Chair in Health and Behaviour at Sinai Health (a joint chair of Sinai Health and the Medical-Psychiatry Alliance of the University of Toronto) and by Sinai Health's Sam and Judy Pencer and Family Chair in Applied General Psychiatry.

Above all, we are profoundly indebted to Isaac for his extraordinary courage in allowing his story to be told for the benefit of others.

Notes

Preface

x ... *affects over sixty million American adults and about nine million Canadian adults*
Childhood adversity that is likely to cause adult health problems occurs in one in
three kids. The evidence for this and a description of what that adversity entails is
detailed in Chapter 2.

1 **"The damage I am"**

2 *A classic paper that called such patients "hateful" ...*
Groves, J. E. (1978). Taking care of the hateful patient. *New England Journal of Medicine, 298,* 883–7.

3 *The idea of ACEs ... comes from a questionnaire that Vincent Felitti and his colleagues developed ...*
Felitti, V. J., Anda, R. F., Nordenberg, D., Williamson, D. F., Spitz, A. M., Edwards,
V., Koss, M. P., & Marks, J. S. (1998). Relationship of childhood abuse and household dysfunction to many of the leading causes of deaths in adults: The adverse
childhood experiences (ACE) study. *American Journal of Preventive Medicine, 14,*
245–58.

3 *We replicated their findings in the family medicine unit at our hospital ...*
Le, T. L., Mann, R. E., Levitan, R. D., George, T. P., & Maunder, R. G. (2017). Sex
differences in the relationships between childhood adversity, attachment anxiety
and current smoking. *Addiction Research & Theory, 25*(2), 146–53.

3 *It's our problem – all of us – not just a problem for "them," whoever they are.*
Although childhood adversity is found everywhere, it is not equally distributed.
Children at increased risk include First Nations, Inuit, and Métis children;
LGBTQ2+ youth; homeless, street-involved youth and youth who misuse drugs; chil-
dren with low socioeconomic status; children who have experienced previous violent

victimization; and immigrant and racialized youth of first-generation and ethnic minorities.

Public Health Agency of Canada. (2019). *Canada's road map to end violence against children.*

3   *Many of the negative mental consequences of ACEs are obvious ...*
Afifi, T. O., MacMillan, H. L., Boyle, M., Taillieu, T., Cheung, K., & Sareen, J. (2014). Child abuse and mental disorders in Canada. *Canadian Medical Association Journal, 186*(9), E324–32.

The US Department of Health and Human Services once estimated that ACEs account for somewhere between one-quarter and one-half of the risk for many of these diseases.

The estimate was made by the National Council for Community Behavioral Healthcare in 2012. The estimate is no longer available online. The calculations that went into this estimate would be valuable to replicate. It is a complicated process to estimate relative proportions of risk attributable to various risk factors. We haven't seen a peer-reviewed paper that estimates the population-attributable risk of the major chronic issues from ACEs, but one is sorely needed.

2   "Fuckin' dead weight"

12   *... the rate of childhood abuse among members of the Canadian military was almost 50 per cent ...*
Afifi, T. O., Taillieu, T., Zamorski, M. A., Turner, S., Cheung, K., & Sareen, J. (2016). Association of child abuse exposure with suicidal ideation, suicide plans, and suicide attempts in military personnel and the general population in Canada. *Journal of the American Medical Association Psychiatry, 73*(3), 229–38.

12   *"sounds like a B.S. study" ...*
Roussy, K. (2016, January 27). *Half of Canadian soldiers faced childhood abuse, study indicates.* CBC News. https://www.cbc.ca/news/health/child-abuse-military-1.3421708

14   *An estimate of the economic burden of reported child maltreatment in the United States found ...*
Peterson, C., Florence, C., & Klevens, J. (2018). The economic burden of child maltreatment in the United States, 2015. *Child Abuse and Neglect, 86,* 178–83.

14   *Using a representative study of these experiences ...*
The definitions that we present and the prevalence of the experiences they describe are from Dr. Traci Afifi's 2014 study. This study used data from the 2012 Canadian Community Health Survey: Mental Health, which was representative of the Canadian population except for excluding residents in the three territories, residents in Indigenous communities, full-time members of the Canadian Forces, and people living in institutions – thus probably underestimating overall rates slightly (the excluded groups constitute about 3 per cent of Canada's population but include people at higher risk). Participants were interviewed by trained lay interviewers using computer-assisted interviewing. The response rate of those asked to participate was high.

Afifi, T. O., MacMillan, H. L., Boyle, M., Taillieu, T., Cheung, K., & Sareen, J. (2014). Child abuse and mental disorders in Canada. *Canadian Medical Association Journal, 186*(9), E324–32.

15 *In his original measure, there were ten categories of ACE events ...*
In the table describing the original ten categories, we have labeled the ten types. The labels are from us, not Felitti.

Felitti, V. J., Anda, R. F., Nordenberg, D., Williamson, D. F., Spitz, A. M., Edwards, V., Koss, M. P., & Marks, J. S. (1998). Relationship of childhood abuse and household dysfunction to many of the leading causes of deaths in adults: The adverse childhood experiences (ACE) study. *American Journal of Preventive Medicine, 14*, 245–58.

The original ACE survey is available through the US Centers for Disease Control and Prevention:

Centers for Disease and Prevention. (2020, April 13). *Violence prevention: CDC Kaiser study.* US Department of Health and Human Services. https://www.cdc.gov /violenceprevention/acestudy/about.html

We put an ACE calculator online, if you would like to see your own ACE score according to the original categories: https://goo.gl/UQDmzX

15 *Almost 60 per cent of people have experienced at least one of the original ten ...*
Felitti, V. J., Anda, R. F., Nordenberg, D., Williamson, D. F., Spitz, A. M., Edwards, V., Koss, M. P., & Marks, J. S. (1998). Relationship of childhood abuse and household dysfunction to many of the leading causes of deaths in adults: The adverse childhood experiences (ACE) study. *American Journal of Preventive Medicine, 14*, 245–58.

Gilbert, L. K., Breiding, M. J., Merrick, M. T., Thompson, W. W., Ford, D. C., Dhingra, S. S., & Parks, S. E. (2015). Childhood adversity and adult chronic disease: An update from ten states and the District of Columbia, 2010. *American Journal of Preventive Medicine, 48*(3), 345–9.

16 *Additional evidence-supported types of childhood adversity ...*
A wider range of categories of ACEs, beyond the original ten, is more realistic and is supported by subsequent research.

Cronholm, P. F., Forke, C. M., Wade, R., Bair-Merritt, M. H., Davis, M., Harkins-Schwarz, M., Pachter, L. M., & Fein, J. A. (2015). Adverse childhood experiences: Expanding the concept of adversity. *American Journal of Preventive Medicine, 49*(3), 354–61.

Finkelhor, D., Shattuck, A., Turner, H., & Hamby, S. (2013). Improving the adverse childhood experiences study scale. *Journal of the American Medical Association Pediatrics, 167*(1), 70–5.

16 *... what child development experts call an invalidating environment.*
Musser, N., Zalewski, M., Stepp, S., & Lewis, J. (2018). A systematic review of negative parenting practices predicting borderline personality disorder: Are we measuring biosocial theory's "invalidating environment"? *Clinical Psychology Review, 65*, 1–16.

3 Drowning

20 *Growing up in an invalidating environment tends to leave a person insecure and mistrustful.*
In this passage, we are describing two fundamental types of attachment insecurity
experienced by adults, according to attachment theory. They are attachment avoidance
(which leads to the distancing response) and attachment anxiety (which leads to depen-
dency). We will allude to attachment theory a few times in this book. For a deeper dive
into those interpersonal patterns and how they affect health and health care, see Maunder, R., & Hunter, J. (2015). *Love, fear, and health: How our attachments to others shape
health and health care.* University of Toronto Press.

22 *"You can tell a true war story if it embarrasses you ...."*
O'Brien, T. (2009). *The things they carried.* Mariner Books.

22 *... an event that feels like having a horse kick you in the gut ...*
We are paraphrasing a description of obstruction by Robert Mason Lee: "First, a
mule is kicking you in the stomach. Second, some maniac is inflating your abdomen
with a bicycle pump. Third, you are being impaled up the ass with a pointy stick.
Still, all comparisons are odious. What it feels like, most of all, is that you are, suddenly, and without warning, very, very sick."
Lee, R. M. (2001, April). The man who was saved by a mouse. *Saturday Night.*

23 *I have never heard a colleague call a patient hateful ...*
Groves, J. E. (1978). Taking care of the hateful patient. *New England Journal of Medicine, 298,* 883–7.

25 *I hate you. Don't leave me.*
This is the title of a book about borderline personality disorder. This personality disorder and the unresolvable tension that comes from disorganized attachment, which
is what we are describing in the passage, are not exactly the same but they overlap.
Kreisman, J. J., & Straus, H. (2010). *I hate you – Don't leave me: Understanding the
borderline personality* (rev. ed.). Tarcher Perigee.

4 "Cure sometimes. Relieve often. Comfort always."

29 *In psychotherapy, the quality of the relationship between the therapist and client is the single
most powerful determinant of good outcomes.*
Norcross, J. C. (2011). *Psychotherapy relations that work: Evidence-based responsiveness*
(2nd ed.). Oxford.

32 *As our population ages, most older people have more than one chronic disease ...*
Pefoyo, A. J., Bronskill, S. E., Gruneir, A., Calzavara, A., Thavorn, K., Petrosyan,
Y., Maxwell, C. J., Bai, Y., & Wodchis, W. P. (2015). The increasing burden and
complexity of multimorbidity. *BMC Public Health, 15,* 415.

32 *When seniors with multiple diseases were interviewed about managing their health ...*
Ploeg, J., Matthew-Maich, N., Fraser, K., Dufour, S., McAiney, C., Kaasalainen,
S., Markle-Reid, M., Upshur, R., Cleghorn, L., & Emili, A. (2017). Managing

multiple chronic conditions in the community: A Canadian qualitative study of the experiences of older adults, family caregivers and healthcare providers. *BMC Geriatrics, 17*(1), 40.

33 *Dr. Lawrence Kirmayer, a psychiatrist at McGill University, calls these unexplained symptoms "a social and clinical predicament, not a specific disorder" ...*
Kirmayer, L. J., Groleau, D., Looper, K. J., & Dao, M. D. (2004). Explaining medically unexplained symptoms. *Canadian Journal of Psychiatry, 49*(10), 663–72.

34 *... five-hundred-year-old folk advice: "Cure sometimes. Relieve often. Comfort always."*
Shaw, Q. (2009). On aphorisms. *British Journal of General Practice, 59*(569), 954–5.

5 "You're in it with me now"

38 *We had one lecture on the "battered child syndrome" ...*
Kempe, C. H., Silverman, F. N., Steele, B. F., Droegemueller, W., & Silver, H. K. (1962). The battered-child syndrome. *Journal of the American Medical Association, 181,* 17–24.

38 *... just about everyone read* The House of God ...
Shem, S. (2010). *The house of God.* Berkley Books.

6 "The closest thing to love"

44 *Neurobiological research is catching up.*
Eisenberger, N. I., Lieberman, M. D., & Williams, K. D. (2003). Does rejection hurt? An FMRI study of social exclusion. *Science, 302*(5643), 290–2.

45 *Thomas Insel, former director of the National Institute of Mental Health ...*
Insel, T. R. (2003). Is social attachment an addictive disorder? *Physiology and Behavior, 79*(3), 351–7.

7 Cause of causes

52 *Comparing the risk of disease between people who had had none ...*
Gilbert, L. K., Breiding, M. J., Merrick, M. T., Thompson, W. W., Ford, D. C., Dhingra, S. S., & Parks, S. E. (2015). Childhood adversity and adult chronic disease: An update from ten states and the District of Columbia, 2010. *American Journal of Preventive Medicine, 48*(3), 345–9.

Afifi, T. O., MacMillan, H. L., Boyle, M., Cheung, K., Taillieu, T., Turner, S., & Sareen, J. (2016). Child abuse and physical health in adulthood. *Health Reports, 27*(3), 10–18.

Fuller-Thomson, E., & Brennenstuhl, S. (2009). Making a link between childhood physical abuse and cancer: Results from a regional representative survey. *Cancer, 115*(14), 3341–50.

53 *In one study, each type of adverse childhood experience on its own increased the likelihood of smoking.*
Ford, E. S., Anda, R. F., Edwards, V. J., Perry, G. S., Zhao, G., Li, C., & Croft, J. B. (2011). Adverse childhood experiences and smoking status in five states. *Preventive Medicine, 53*(3), 188–93.

54 *A survey of thousands of adults in Washington State found that those who experienced childhood sexual abuse were ...*
Bensley, L. S., Van Eenwyk, J., & Simmons, K. W. (2000). Self-reported childhood sexual and physical abuse and adult HIV-risk behaviors and heavy drinking. *American Journal of Preventive Medicine, 18*(2), 151–8.

54 *One study found that those with ACE scores of six or more died twenty years younger ...*
Brown, D. W., Anda, R. F., Tiemeier, H., Felitti, V. J., Edwards, V. J., Croft, J. B., & Giles, W. H. (2009). Adverse childhood experiences and the risk of premature mortality. *American Journal of Preventive Medicine, 37*(5), 389–96.

54 *... childhood adversity leads to "radically different life-course trajectories."*
Bellis, M. A., Hughes, K., Leckenby, N., Hardcastle, K. A., Perkins, C., & Lowey, H. (2015). Measuring mortality and the burden of adult disease associated with adverse childhood experiences in England: A national survey. *Journal of Public Health (Oxford, England), 37*(3), 445–54.

54 *... the health burden of smoking more, drinking more, and other risky behaviors doesn't account for all of this early mortality.*
Kelly-Irving, M., Lepage, B., Dedieu, D., Bartley, M., Blane, D., Grosclaude, P., Lang, T., & Delpierre, C. (2013). Adverse childhood experiences and premature all-cause mortality. *European Journal of Epidemiology, 28*(9), 721–4.

54 *This can be measured by the length of telomeres ...*
Kiecolt-Glaser, J. K., Gouin, J. P., Weng, N. P., Malarkey, W. B., Beversdorf, D. Q., & Glaser, R. (2011). Childhood adversity heightens the impact of later-life caregiving stress on telomere length and inflammation. *Psychosomatic Medicine, 73*(1), 16–22.
Shalev, I., Moffitt, T. E., Sugden, K., Williams, B., Houts, R. M., Danese, A., Mill, J., Arseneault, L., & Caspi, A. (2013). Exposure to violence during childhood is associated with telomere erosion from 5 to 10 years of age: A longitudinal study. *Molecular Psychiatry, 18*(5), 576–81.

58 *Importantly, health care providers may not even be considered reliable sources of knowledge ...*
This construct, known as epistemic distrust, is common among people with unexplained physical symptoms and functional syndromes and profoundly complicates their medical care.
Luyten, P., & De Meulemeester, C. (2017). Understanding and treatment of patients with persistent somatic complaints through the lens of contemporary attachment theory. *Attachment, 11*(3), 205–22.

8 "Speak for me"

62 *"Listen to the patient, he is telling you the diagnosis," said Dr. William Osler.*
The origin of the quote is uncertain, but it is widely attributed to Osler.

Silverman, M. E., Murray, T. J., & Bryan, C. S. (Eds.). (2003). *The quotable Osler.* American College of Physicians.

62 *A classic study found that when doctors speak with patients, on average they interrupt them in about eighteen seconds.*
Beckman, H. B., & Frankel, R. M. (1984). The effect of physician behavior on the collection of data. *Annals of Internal Medicine, 101,* 692–6.

62 *... we have our interrupting time down to eleven seconds now.*
Singh Ospina, N., Phillips, K. A., Rodriguez-Gutierrez, R., Castaneda-Guarderas, A., Gionfriddo, M. R., Branda, M. E., & Montori, V. M. (2019). Eliciting the patient's agenda – Secondary analysis of recorded clinical encounters. *Journal of General Internal Medicine, 34*(1), 36–40.

63 *Trauma leads to narrative incoherence.*
The construct of narrative coherence and incoherence that we are referring to is from adult attachment theory, particularly from the usual method of identifying different categories of attachment, the Adult Attachment Interview (AAI). The link between attachment and developmental trauma is strong, with unresolved trauma corresponding to the most severe category of insecure attachment, disorganized attachment, which would certainly be Isaac's category (technically, he would be both dismissing and disorganized).

In the AAI, people are asked quite challenging questions about emotional aspects of their closest relationships, especially while growing up, and then transcripts of their responses are assessed in several ways, including for their linguistic characteristics according to Grice's four maxims of quality (have evidence for what you say), quantity (be succinct yet complete), relation (be relevant to the topic at hand), and manner (be clear and orderly). We learned of many of the specific qualities of speech choices related to Isaac's style (dismissing) and to the other style described below it (preoccupied) while training in interpretation of the Adult Attachment Projective System, a descendant of the AAI, developed by Carol George and Malcolm West.

Daniel, S. I. (2009). The developmental roots of narrative expression in therapy: Contributions from attachment theory and research. *Psychotherapy, 46*(3), 301–16.

George, C., & West, M. L. (2012). *The adult attachment projective picture system.* Guilford Press.

Hesse, E. (2008). The Adult Attachment Interview: Protocol, method of analysis, and empirical studies. In J. Cassidy & P. R. Shaver (Eds.), *Handbook of attachment: Theory, research and clinical applications* (2nd ed., pp. 552–98). Guilford Press.

64 *Technically, when the story's audience is just one person, this is called* mentalizing ...
Luyten, P., & Fonagy, P. (2015). The neurobiology of mentalizing. *Personality Disorders, 6*(4), 366–79.

Markowitz, J. C., Milrod, B., Luyten, P., & Holmqvist, R. (2019). Mentalizing in interpersonal psychotherapy. *American Journal of Psychotherapy, 72*(4), 95–100.

9 Fever

69 *"the patient is the one with the disease."*
Shem, S. (2010). *The house of God.* Berkley Books.

69 *We find that childhood trauma is just as common among people who work in hospitals ...*
Maunder, R. G., Peladeau, N., Savage, D., & Lancee, W. J. (2010). The prevalence of childhood adversity among healthcare workers and its relationship to adult life events, distress and impairment. *Child Abuse and Neglect, 34*(2), 114–23.

69 *For some first responders, the rates are much higher ...*
Maunder, R. G., Halpern, J., Schwartz, B., & Gurevich, M. (2012). Symptoms and responses to critical incidents in paramedics who have experienced childhood abuse and neglect. *Emergency Medicine Journal, 29*(3), 222–7.

70 *Nurses are exposed to physical and emotional abuse alarmingly frequently.*
A review of studies of over one hundred and fifty thousand nurses found that more than a third reported exposure to workplace physical violence and often were injured.
Spector, P. E., Zhou, Z. E., & Che, X. X. (2014). Nurse exposure to physical and nonphysical violence, bullying, and sexual harassment: A quantitative review. *International Journal of Nursing Studies, 51*(1), 72–84.

70 *Suicide rates are elevated in female physicians and in some specialties, such as psychiatry and anesthesia ...*
Duarte, D., El-Hagrassy, M. M., Couto, T. C. E., Gurgel, W., Fregni, F., & Correa, H. (2020). Male and female physician suicidality: A systematic review and meta-analysis. *Journal of the American Medical Association Psychiatry, 77*(6), 587–97.

70 *Burnout ... affecting between a quarter and a third of health care professionals.*
Dyrbye, L. N., West, C. P., Satele, D., Boone, S., Tan, L., Sloan, J., & Shanafelt, T. D. (2014). Burnout among US medical students, residents, and early career physicians relative to the general US population. *Academic Medicine: Journal of the Association of American Medical Colleges, 89*(3), 443–51.

Monsalve-Reyes, C. S., San Luis-Costas, C., Gomez-Urquiza, J. L., Albendin-Garcia, L., Aguayo, R., & Canadas-De la Fuente, G. A. (2018). Burnout syndrome and its prevalence in primary care nursing: A systematic review and meta-analysis. *BMC Family Practice, 19*(1), 59.

Soler, J. K., Yaman, H., Esteva, M., Dobbs, F., Asenova, R. S., Katic, M., Ozvacic, Z., Desgranges, J. P., Moreau, A., Lionis, C., Kotányi, P., Carelli, F., Nowak, P. R., de Aguiar Sá Azeredo, Z., Marklund, E., Churchill, D., Ungan, M., & European General Practice Research Network Burnout Study Group. (2008). Burnout in European family doctors: The EGPRN study. *Family Practice, 25*(4), 245–65.

Trufelli, D. C., Bensi, C. G., Garcia, J. B., Narahara, J. L., Abrão, M. N., Diniz, R. W., Miranda, V., Soares, H. P., & Del Giglio, A. (2008). Burnout in cancer professionals: a systematic review and meta-analysis. *European Journal of Cancer Care, 17*(6), 524–31.

70 *... burnout about doubles the odds that a physician will be involved in a "patient safety incident."*

Panagioti, M., Panagopoulou, E., Bower, P., Lewith, G., Kontopantelis, E., Chew-Graham, C., Dawson, S., van Marwijk, H., Geraghty, K., & Esmail, A. (2017). Controlled interventions to reduce burnout in physicians: A systematic review and meta-analysis. *Journal of the American Medical Association Internal Medicine*, 177(2), 195–205.

71 *Patients understand that the question is relevant and don't mind being asked as long as it is done in a way that feels safe and respectful ...*
Berry, K. M., & Rutledge, C. M. (2016). Factors that influence women to disclose sexual assault history to health care providers. *Journal of Obstetric, Gynecologic, and Neonatal Nursing*, 45(4), 553–64.

Gillespie, R. J., & Folger, A. T. (2017). Feasibility of assessing parental ACEs in pediatric primary care: Implications for practice-based implementation. *Journal of Child & Adolescent Trauma*, 10(3), 249–56.

Schachter, C. L., Radomsky, N. A., Stalker, C. A., & Teram, E. (2004). Women survivors of child sexual abuse. How can health professionals promote healing? *Canadian Family Physician*, 50, 405–12.

71 *Some doctors, particularly the younger ones, appreciate that they should ask, but mostly don't.*
Friedman, L. S., Samet, J. H., Roberts, M. S., Hudlin, M., & Hans, P. (1992). Inquiry about victimization experiences. A survey of patient preferences and physician practices. *Archives of Internal Medicine*, 152(6), 1186–90.

Maunder, R. G., Hunter, J. J., Tannenbaum, D. W., Le, T. L., & Lay, C. (2020). Physicians' knowledge and practices regarding screening adult patients for adverse childhood experiences: A survey. *BMC Health Services Research*, 20(1), 314.

Tink, W., Tink, J. C., Turin, T. C., & Kelly, M. (2017). Adverse childhood experiences: Survey of resident practice, knowledge, and attitude. *Family Medicine*, 49(1), 7–13.

71 *A survey of doctors that we conducted suggested their behavior depends on their specialty.*
Maunder, R. G., Hunter, J. J., Tannenbaum, D. W., Le, T. L., & Lay, C. (2020). Physicians' knowledge and practices regarding screening adult patients for adverse childhood experiences: A survey. *BMC Health Services Research*, 20(1), 314.

10 Partialists

78 *... by the time you've tried two or three, there is a diminishing return ...*
Gaynes, B. N., Warden, D., Trivedi, M. H., Wisniewski, S. R., Fava, M., & Rush, A. J. (2009). What did STAR*D teach us? Results from a large-scale, practical, clinical trial for patients with depression. *Psychiatric Services*, 60(11), 1439–45.

12 Gifts

90 *Doing therapy with someone who has been sexually abused often raises challenges ...*
Norris, D. M., Gutheil, T. G., & Strasburger, L. H. (2003). This couldn't happen to me: Boundary problems and sexual misconduct in the psychotherapy relationship. *Psychiatric Services*, 54(4), 517–22.

13 "It ends here"

99 *The clearest evidence of this is from crimes against humanity ...*
Bombay, A., Matheson, K., & Anisman, H. (2011). The impact of stressors on second generation Indian residential school survivors. *Transcultural Psychiatry, 48*(4), 367–91.

Bombay, A., Matheson, K., & Anisman, H. (2014). The intergenerational effects of Indian residential schools: Implications for the concept of historical trauma. *Transcultural Psychiatry, 51*(3), 320–38.

Hackett, C., Feeny, D., & Tompa, E. (2016). Canada's residential school system: Measuring the intergenerational impact of familial attendance on health and mental health outcomes. *Journal of Epidemiology and Community Health, 70*(11), 1096–105.

Lee, J., Kwak, Y. S., Kim, Y. J., Kim, E. J., Park, E. J., Shin, Y., Lee, B. H., Lee, S. H., Jung, H. Y., Lee, I., Hwang, J. I., Kim, D., & Lee, S. I. (2019). Transgenerational transmission of trauma: Psychiatric evaluation of offspring of former "comfort women," survivors of the Japanese military sexual slavery during World War II. *Psychiatry Investigation, 16*(3), 249–53.

McQuaid, R. J., Bombay, A., McInnis, O. A., Humeny, C., Matheson, K., & Anisman, H. (2017). Suicide ideation and attempts among First Nations Peoples living on-reserve in Canada: The intergenerational and cumulative effects of Indian residential schools. *Canadian Journal of Psychiatry, 62*(6), 422–30.

100 *Among her several studies exploring the intergenerational effects of the Indian residential school system in Canada ...*
Bombay, A., Matheson, K., & Anisman, H. (2014). Appraisals of discriminatory events among adult offspring of Indian residential school survivors: The influences of identity centrality and past perceptions of discrimination. *Cultural Diversity & Ethnic Minority Psychology, 20*(1), 75–86.

Yehuda, R., Halligan, S. L., & Grossman, R. (2001). Childhood trauma and risk for PTSD: Relationship to intergenerational effects of trauma, parental PTSD, and cortisol excretion. *Development and Psychopathology, 13*(3), 733–53.

100 *In both the survivors of the Holocaust and their children, regulation of genes ...*
Yehuda, R., Daskalakis, N. P., Bierer, L. M., Bader, H. N., Klengel, T., Holsboer, F., & Binder, E. B. (2016). Holocaust exposure induced intergenerational effects on FKBP5 methylation. *Biological Psychiatry, 80*(5), 372–80.

101 *Among perpetrators of child sexual abuse, the likelihood they themselves ...*
Glasser, M., Kolvin, I., Campbell, D., Glasser, A., Leitch, I., & Farrelly, S. (2001). Cycle of child sexual abuse: Links between being a victim and becoming a perpetrator. *British Journal of Psychiatry, 179*, 482–94; discussion 495–7.

Jespersen, A. F., Lalumiere, M. L., & Seto, M. C. (2009). Sexual abuse history among adult sex offenders and non-sex offenders: A meta-analysis. *Child Abuse and Neglect, 33*(3), 179–92.

Whitaker, D. J., Le, B., Karl Hanson, R., Baker, C. K., McMahon, P. M., Ryan, G., Klein, A., & Rice, D. D. (2008). Risk factors for the perpetration of child sexual abuse: A review and meta-analysis. *Child Abuse and Neglect, 32*(5), 529–48.

14 "Help me"

105 *Most children keep it to themselves ...*
McElvaney, R. (2015). Disclosure of child sexual abuse: Delays, non-disclosure and partial disclosure. What the research tells us and implications for practice. *Child Abuse Review, 24*(3), 159–69.

106 *Unsurprisingly, but unfortunately, the more severe the experience of sexual abuse, the less likely a child will speak to an adult.*
Priebe, G., & Svedin, C. G. (2008). Child sexual abuse is largely hidden from the adult society. An epidemiological study of adolescents' disclosures. *Child Abuse and Neglect, 32*(12), 1095–108.

106 *It doesn't have to be that way.*
McElvaney, R. (2015). Disclosure of child sexual abuse: Delays, non-disclosure and partial disclosure. What the research tells us and implications for practice. *Child Abuse Review, 24*(3), 159–69.

Jobe, A., & Gorin, S. (2013). "If kids don't feel safe they don't do anything": Young people's views on seeking and receiving help from Children's Social Care Services in England. *Child & Family Social Work, 18*(4), 429–38.

106 *It isn't just kids. As adults, men who were sexually abused as boys silence themselves or feel silenced.*
Easton, S. D., Saltzman, L. Y., & Willis, D. G. (2014). "Would you tell under circumstances like that?": Barriers to disclosure of child sexual abuse for men. *Psychology of Men & Masculinity, 15*(4), 460–9.

106 *Women are similarly reluctant to speak about sexual violence, expecting, for good reason, to be blamed or not to be believed.*
Fisher, B. S., Daigle, L. E., Cullen, F. T., & Turner, M. G. (2003). Reporting sexual victimization to the police and others: Results from a national-level study of college women. *Criminal Justice and Behavior, 30*(1), 6–38.

106 *There are even more barriers for people of color who experience discrimination and for immigrants ...*
Bauer, H. M., Rodriguez, M. A., Quiroga, S. S., & Flores-Ortiz, Y. G. (2000). Barriers to health care for abused Latina and Asian immigrant women. *Journal of Health Care for the Poor and Underserved, 11*(1), 33–44.

Bonomi, A. E., Holt, V. L., Martin, D. P., & Thompson, R. S. (2006). Severity of intimate partner violence and occurrence and frequency of police calls. *Journal of Interpersonal Violence, 21*(10), 1354–64.

Hien, D., & Ruglass, L. (2009). Interpersonal partner violence and women in the United States: An overview of prevalence rates, psychiatric correlates and consequences and barriers to help seeking. *International Journal of Law and Psychiatry, 32*(1), 48–55.

Naved, R. T., Azim, S., Bhuiya, A., & Persson, L. A. (2006). Physical violence by husbands: Magnitude, disclosure and help seeking behavior of women in Bangladesh. *Social Science and Medicine, 62*(12), 2917–29.

Roberts, A. L., Gilman, S. E., Breslau, J., Breslau, N., & Koenen, K. C. (2011). Race/ethnic differences in exposure to traumatic events, development of

post-traumatic stress disorder, and treatment-seeking for post-traumatic stress disorder in the United States. *Psychological Medicine, 41*(1), 71–83.

Sabina, C., Cuevas, C. A., & Schally, J. L. (2012). Help-seeking in a national
sample of victimized Latino women: The influence of victimization types. *Journal of
Interpersonal Violence, 27*(1), 40–61.

Ullman, S. E., & Brecklin, L. R. (2002). Sexual assault history and suicidal behavior in a national sample of women. *Suicide & Life-Threatening Behavior, 32*(2), 117–30.

15 Under siege

116 *One psychotherapy expert, Jon Allen, playfully calls it plain old therapy (POT).*
Allen, J. G. (2013). *Restoring mentalizing in attachment relationships: Treating trauma
with plain old therapy.* American Psychiatric Publishing.

117 *"And then, I think of the stages of coping ..."*
We teach, and often rely on, an approach to coping that is adapted from a model
proposed by Susan Folkman and Steven Greer. They drew upon the best evidence
available at the time to describe a model of coping with cancer, but the framework
applies to much more than cancer. In fact, we described a version of our adaptation in a YouTube video called *How to Cope with Anything Including COVID-19* to
help our colleagues with the pandemic.

The gist of the model is straightforward. There are three stages that are used in
sequence. The first is problem-based coping; try to fix the things that you can. That
involves things like planning, learning, breaking big problems down into smaller
ones, considering options, and acting to solve the problem. Second is emotion-
based coping; if you can't fix it, then do things that make you feel better in spite
of an unsolvable problem. This stage emphasizes various kinds of self-care, stress
reduction, and distraction. The third phase, and so the least frequently invoked, is
meaning-based coping. Do things that allow you to reflect on the things that give
you purpose and give your life meaning. The third stage is what is usually used to
cope with enduring suffering.

Folkman, S., & Greer, S. (2000). Promoting psychological well-being in the face
of serious illness: When theory, research and practice inform each other. *Psycho-
Oncology, 9,* 11–19.

Maunder, R., & Hunter, J. (2020, April 2). *Three steps to coping with anything
including COVID-19* [Video]. YouTube. https://youtu.be/ipO3AuqbZq8

121 *These specific elements ...*
Another 15 per cent of the benefits of therapy are attributed to expecting to
improve (placebo effects) while 40 per cent is due to other stuff that has nothing
to do with therapy (like life getting better). Those are statistics that should lead
therapists to try to be decent people (common factors) and to have a great deal of
humility about their expertise.

Norcross, J. C. (2011). *Psychotherapy relations that work: Evidence-based responsiveness*
(2nd ed.). Oxford.

121 *The common factors are ...*
Leszcz, M., Pain, C., Hunter, J., Maunder, R., & Ravitz, P. (2015). *Psychotherapy essentials to go: Achieving psychotherapy effectiveness.* WW Norton & Company.

121 *Clients of effective therapists are twice as likely to get better ...*
Baldwin, S. A., & Imel, Z. E. (2013). Therapist effects: Findings and methods. In M. J. Lambert (Ed.), *Bergin and Garfield's handbook of psychotherapy and behavior changes* (6th ed.). John Wiley & Sons.

16 "Boohoo"

126 *"the traditional first step in the time-honored barbarism required to produce an English gentleman"*
Holmes, J. (2014). *John Bowlby and attachment theory* (2nd ed.). Taylor and Francis.

127 *But Bowlby also recognized there was a common variant of compulsive self-reliance that he called* compulsive caregiving.
Bowlby, J. (1980). *Attachment and loss. Vol. 3: Loss: Sadness and depression.* Basic Books, p. 156.

17 Running

134 *Men who are dismissing and self-reliant, like Isaac, have each of these tests less often than other men.*
Considine, N. S., Tuck, N. L., & Fiori, K. L. (2013). Attachment and health care utilization among middle-aged and older African-descent men: Dismissiveness predicts less frequent digital rectal examination and prostate-specific antigen screening. *American Journal of Men's Health, 7*(5), 382–93. https://doi.org/10.1177/1557988312474838

134 *Same thing for women regarding breast self-examination and mammograms.*
Tuck, N. L., & Considine, N. S. (2015). Breast cancer screening: The role of attachment. *Psychology, Health, and Medicine, 20*(4), 400–9.

134 *It is a blood test that summarizes how well they have controlled their blood sugar levels over the previous three months.*
Glycated hemoglobin is reported as the percentage of hemoglobin molecules that have undergone a chemical change ("become glycated") as a result of being bathed in the sugar that circulates in the bloodstream. Each decrease in HbA1c by 1 per cent cuts the risk of complications in the kidneys, nerves, and eyes by about 25 per cent.
     Stratton, I. M., Adler, A. I., Neil, H. A., Matthews, D. R., Manley, S. E., Cull, C. A., Hadden, D., Turner, R. C., & Holman, R. R. (2000). Association of glycaemia with macrovascular and microvascular complications of type 2 diabetes (UKPDS 35): Prospective observational study. *British Medical Journal, 321*(7258), 405–12.

134 *People with Isaac's interpersonal style ... have substantially higher HbA1c than all others ...*
Ciechanowski, P. S., Katon, W. J., Russo, J. E., & Walker, E. A. (2001). The patient-provider relationship: Attachment theory and adherence to treatment in diabetes. *American Journal of Psychiatry, 158*(1), 29–35.

18 "Who is going to give a shit?"

138 *She interviewed patients who struggle with symptoms, as Isaac does, or with health anxiety and she talked to their family doctors.*
Le, T. L., Mylopoulos, M., Bearss, E., Geist, R., & Maunder, R. (2021). Physical symptoms and health anxiety in primary care: A qualitative study of tensions and collaboration between patients and family doctors. (Submitted for publication)

19 "I've got this figured out"

145 *Trauma-informed care attends to many kinds of violence and trauma …*
Elliott, D. E., Bjelajac, P., Fallot, R. D., Markoff, L. S., & Reed, B. G. (2005). Trauma-informed or trauma-denied: Principles and implementation of trauma-informed services for women. *Journal of Community Psychology, 33*(3), 461–7.
Harris, M., & Fallot, R. D. (Eds.). (2001). *Using trauma-informed theory to design service systems.* Jossey-Bass/Wiley.

20 "I used to think that nothing could change"

151 *As we have argued elsewhere …*
Maunder, R. G., & Hunter, J. J. (2017, May 30). How childhood trauma can lead to chronic illness. *The Walrus.* https://thewalrus.ca/how-childhood-trauma-can-lead-to-chronic-illness/

21 The Care Revolution

153 *We have stacks of reports, guidelines, and road maps …*
Center for Disease Control and Prevention. (n.d.). *Child abuse and neglect prevention strategies.* US Department of Health and Human Services. https://www.cdc.gov/violenceprevention/childabuseandneglect/prevention.html
Hendrikson, H., & Blackman, K. (2015, August). *State policies addressing child abuse and neglect.* National Conference of State Legislatures. https://www.ncsl.org/Portals/1/Documents/Health/StatePolicies_ChildAbuse.pdf
Office for the Victims of Crime. (n.d.). *Initiatives to combat child abuse.* US Department of Justice, Office of Justice Programs. https://www.ncjrs.gov/ovc_archives/factsheets/childabu.htm
Children's Bureau. (2018, December 24). *Child abuse & neglect.* Administration for Children and Families, US Department of Health and Human Services. https://www.acf.hhs.gov/cb/focus-areas/child-abuse-neglect
Substance Abuse and Mental Health Services Administration Trauma and Justice Strategic Initiative. (2014, July). *SAMHSA's concept of trauma and guidance for a*

trauma-informed approach. US Department of Health and Human Services. https:// ncsacw.samhsa.gov/userfiles/files/SAMHSA_Trauma.pdf

Menschner, C., & Maul, A. (2016, April). *Issue brief: Key ingredients for successful trauma-informed care implementation.* Center for Health Care Strategies. https://www .traumainformedcare.chcs.org/wp-content/uploads/2018/11/Brief-Key-Ingredients -for-TIC-Implementation.pdf

World Health Organization. (2021). *Inspire: Seven strategies for ending violence against children.* https://www.who.int/violence_injury_prevention/violence/inspire -package/en/

Public Health Agency of Canada. (2019, July 15). *Canada's road map to end violence against children.* https://www.canada.ca/en/public-health/services /publications/healthy-living/road-map-end-violence-against-children.html

154 ... *the CARE method of asking about childhood adversity.*
Maunder, R. (2019, November 28). *The CARE method of screening ACEs: How and why to ask adult patients about childhood adversity* [Video]. YouTube. https://youtu.be /fc7NBdCYUAE

166 *During their medical training, most of them will become* less *empathic.*
Ferreira-Valente, A., Monteiro, J. S., Barbosa, R. M., Salgueira, A., Costa, P., & Costa, M. J. (2017). Clarifying changes in student empathy throughout medical school: A scoping review. *Advances in Health Sciences Education: Theory and Practice,* 22(5), 1293-313.

166 *An alarming number of them will be showing signs of professional burnout before they have even acquired a license to treat patients. Some will even die by suicide.*
Dyrbye, L. N., West, C. P., Satele, D., Boone, S., Tan, L., Sloan, J., & Shanafelt, T. D. (2014). Burnout among US medical students, residents, and early career physicians relative to the general US population. *Academic Medicine: Journal of the Association of American Medical Colleges,* 89(3), 443-51.

Rubin R. (2014). Recent suicides highlight need to address depression in medical students and residents. *Journal of the American Medical Association, 312*(17), 1725-7.

166 *At some medical schools, cases have been developed expressly to introduce trauma-informed care ...*
Pletcher, B. A., O'Connor, M., Swift-Taylor, M. E., & DallaPiazza, M. (2019). Adverse childhood experiences: A case-based workshop introducing medical students to trauma-informed care. *MedEdPORTAL, 15,* 10803.

Elisseou, S., Puranam, S., & Nandi, M. (2018). A novel, trauma-informed physical examination curriculum. *Medical Education, 52*(5), 555-6.

167 *We have a great deal to review, discuss, and apply, from the scientific statement of the American Heart Association ...*
See the evidence cited in Chapter 7. The American Heart Association scientific statement is found here:

Suglia, S. F., Koenen, K. C., Boynton-Jarrett, R., Chan, P. S., Clark, C. J., Danese, A., Faith, M. S., Goldstein, B. I., Hayman, L. L., Isasi, C. R., Pratt, C. A.,

Slopen, N., Sumner, J. A., Turer, A., Turer, C. B., Zachariah, J. P., American Heart Association Council on Epidemiology and Prevention, Council on Cardiovascular Disease in the Young, Council on Functional Genomics and Translational Biology, Council on Cardiovascular and Stroke Nursing, & Council on Quality of Care and Outcomes Research. (2018). Childhood and adolescent adversity and cardio-metabolic outcomes: A scientific statement from the American Heart Association. *Circulation, 137*(5), e15–e28. https://doi.org/10.1161/CIR.0000000000000536

167 *They need to practice difficult interactions, which is best accomplished through encounters with simulated patients who are observed and coached.*

Ravitz, P., Lancee, W. J., Lawson, A., Maunder, R., Hunter, J. J., Leszcz, M., McNaughton, N., & Pain, C. (2013). Improving physician-patient communication through coaching of simulated encounters. *Academic Psychiatry, 37*(2), 87–93.

168 *One way to accelerate change is to link the revolution in trauma-informed care to comple-mentary disruptive forces from anti-racist, feminist, and queer perspectives ...*

Sharma, M. (2019). Applying feminist theory to medical education. *Lancet, 393*(10171), 570–8.

Hardeman, R. R., Burgess, D., Murphy, K., Satin, D. J., Nielsen, J., Potter, T. M., Karbeah, J., Zulu-Gillespie, M., Apolinario-Wilcoxon, A., Reif, C., & Cunningham, B. A. (2018). Developing a medical school curriculum on racism: Multi-disciplinary, multiracial conversations informed by public health critical race praxis (PHCRP). *Ethnicity & Disease, 28*(Suppl 1), 271–8.

Phelan, S. M., Burke, S. E., Cunningham, B. A., Perry, S. P., Hardeman, R. R., Dovidio, J. F., Herrin, J., Dyrbye, L. N., White, R. O., Yeazel, M. W., Onyeador, I. N., Wittlin, N. M., Harden, K., & van Ryn, M. (2019). The effects of racism in medical education on students' decisions to practice in underserved or minority communities. *Academic Medicine : Journal of the Association of American Medical Colleges, 94*(8), 1178–89.

Cooper, M. B., Chacko, M., & Christner, J. (2018). Incorporating LGBT health in an undergraduate medical education curriculum through the construct of social determinants of health. *MedEdPORTAL, 14*, 10781.

Robertson, W. J. (2017). The irrelevance narrative: Queer (in)visibility in medical education and practice. *Medical Anthropology Quarterly, 31*(2), 159–76.

172 *"... child welfare organizations are trying to make these changes, but everyone is 'choosing their own adventure.'"*

One useful approach to organizational change toward trauma-informed care was developed by Trauma Informed Oregon, which is a collaboration between the Oregon Health Authority, Health Systems Division, and Portland State University, in partnership with Oregon Health & Science University and the Oregon Pediatric Society.

Trauma Informed Oregon website: https://traumainformedoregon.org

173 *The Circle of Security program ...*

Hoffman, K. T., Marvin, R. S., Cooper, G., & Powell, B. (2006). Changing toddlers' and preschoolers' attachment classifications: The Circle of Security intervention. *Journal of Consulting and Clinical Psychology, 74*(6), 1017–26.

173 *The Nurse-Family Partnership ...*

Olds, D. L., Henderson, C. R., Jr., & Kitzman, H. (1994). Does prenatal and infancy nurse home visitation have enduring effects on qualities of parental caregiving and child health at 25 to 50 months of life? *Pediatrics, 93*(1), 89–98.

Olds, D. L., Kitzman, H., Cole, R., Robinson, J., Sidora, K., Luckey, D. W., Henderson, C. R., Jr., Hanks, C., Bondy, J., & Holmberg, J. (2004). Effects of nurse home-visiting on maternal life course and child development: Age 6 follow-up results of a randomized trial. *Pediatrics, 114*(6), 1550–9.

Olds, D. L., Kitzman, H., Knudtson, M. D., Anson, E., Smith, J. A., & Cole, R. (2014). Effect of home visiting by nurses on maternal and child mortality: Results of a 2-decade follow-up of a randomized clinical trial. *Journal of the American Medical Association Pediatrics, 168*(9), 800–6.

Nurse-Family Partnership website: https://www.nursefamilypartnership.org

174 *... the Attachment Biobehavioral Catch-Up (ABC) program ...*

Bernard, K., Dozier, M., Bick, J., Lewis-Morrarty, E., Lindhiem, O., & Carlson, E. (2012). Enhancing attachment organization among maltreated children: Results of a randomized clinical trial. *Child Development, 83*(2), 623–36.

Dozier, M., Peloso, E., Lindhiem, O., Gordon, M. K., Manni, M., Sepulveda, S., Ackerman, J., Bernier, A., & Levine, S. (2006). Developing evidence-based interventions for foster children: An example of a randomized clinical trial with infants and toddlers. *Journal of Social Issues, 62,* 767–85.

The ABC website: http://www.abcintervention.org

175 *... there is compelling evidence that psychiatrists who see the same patients for many years ... create a barrier ...*

Kurdyak, P., Stukel, T. A., Goldbloom, D., Kopp, A., Zagorski, B. M., & Mulsant, B. H. (2014). Universal coverage without universal access: A study of psychiatrist supply and practice patterns in Ontario. *Open Medicine, 8*(3), e87–e99.

Kurdyak, P., Zaheer, J., Carvalho, A., de Oliveira, C., Lebenbaum, M., Wilton, A. S., Fefergrad, M., Stergiopoulos, V., & Mulsant, B. H. (2020). Physician-based availability of psychotherapy in Ontario: A population-based retrospective cohort study. *Canadian Medical Association Journal Open, 8*(1), E105–15.

175 *High-quality psychotherapy is an effective treatment for many mental illnesses, including most of those caused by childhood adversity.*

Duberstein, P. R., Ward, E. A., Chaudron, L. H., He, H., Toth, S. L., Wang, W., Van Orden, K. A., Gamble, S. A., & Talbot, N. L. (2018). Effectiveness of interpersonal psychotherapy-trauma for depressed women with childhood abuse histories. *Journal of Consulting and Clinical Psychology, 86*(10), 868–78.

Munder, T., Fluckiger, C., Leichsenring, F., Abbass, A. A., Hilsenroth, M. J., Luyten, P., Rabung, S., Steinert, C., & Wampold, B. E. (2019). Is psychotherapy effective? A re-analysis of treatments for depression. *Epidemiology and Psychiatric Sciences, 28*(3), 268–74.

Tasca, G. A., Town, J. M., Abbass, A., & Clarke, J. (2018). Will publicly funded psychotherapy in Canada be evidence based? A review of what makes psychotherapy work and a proposal. *Canadian Psychology, 59*(4), 293–300.

Watkins, L. E., Sprang, K. R., & Rothbaum, B. O. (2018). Treating PTSD: A review of evidence-based psychotherapy interventions. *Frontiers in Behavioral Neuroscience, 12*, 258.

175 *In 2012, a lack of counseling was the most frequent unmet need of Canadians with mental health challenges ...*
Sunderland, A., & Findlay, L. C. (2013). Perceived need for mental health care in Canada: Results from the 2012 Canadian Community Health Survey-Mental Health. *Health Reports, 24*(9), 3–9.

175 *... access [to psychotherapy] was worse for those with lower incomes.*
Bartram, M., & Stewart, J. M. (2019). Income-based inequities in access to psychotherapy and other mental health services in Canada and Australia. *Health Policy, 123*(1), 45–50.

175 *In the United States, the economics of health care are very different, but problems with access to mental health care are similar.*
Kliff, S. (2012, December 17). Seven facts about America's mental health-care system. *Washington Post.* https://www.washingtonpost.com/news/wonk/wp/2012/12/17/seven-facts-about-americas-mental-health-care-system/

175 *It is worse for Mexican Americans, Black people, and presumably other racialized people.*
Gonzalez, H. M., Vega, W. A., Williams, D. R., Tarraf, W., West, B. T., & Neighbors, H. W. (2010). Depression care in the United States: Too little for too few. *Archives of General Psychiatry, 67*(1), 37–46.

176 *The United Kingdom has demonstrated a way forward by putting a massive effort into implementing a model called Increased Access to Psychotherapy ...*
Gratzer, D., & Goldbloom, D. (2016). Making evidence-based psychotherapy more accessible in Canada. *Canadian Journal of Psychiatry, 61*(10), 618–23.

Clark, D. M., Canvin, L., Green, J., Layard, R., Pilling, S., & Janecka, M. (2018). Transparency about the outcomes of mental health services (IAPT approach): An analysis of public data. *Lancet, 391*(10121), 679–6.

176 *Heather has gained so much experience supporting Derek as his partner that she now provides resources and education to other partners in her position*
Heather Tuba website: https://heathertuba.com

181 *By 2019, just nine of the ninety-four calls had been implemented.*
Jewell, E., & Mosby, I. (2019, December 17). *Calls to action accountability: A status update on reconciliation.* Yellowhead Institute. https://yellowheadinstitute.org/2019/12/17/calls-to-action-accountability-a-status-update-on-reconciliation/

181 *Dr. Tracie Afifi ... cites twenty years of research that demonstrates "that spanking is associated with an increased probability of mental health problems ..."*
Afifi, T. O., & Romano, E. (2017). Ending the spanking debate. *Child Abuse and Neglect, 71*, 3–4.

See also Afifi, T. O., Ford, D., Gershoff, E. T., Merrick, M., Grogan-Kaylor, A., Ports, K. A., MacMillan, H. L., Holden, G. W., Taylor, C. A., Lee, S. J., & Peters Bennett, R. (2017). Spanking and adult mental health impairment: The case for the designation of spanking as an adverse childhood experience. *Child Abuse and Neglect, 71,* 24–31.
182 *In 2016, 57 per cent of Canadians regarded spanking a child as "always or usually morally wrong."*
Barnett, L. (2016, June 3). *The "spanking" law: Section 43 of the Criminal Code* (Publication No. 2016-35-E). Legal and Social Affairs Division, Parliamentary Information and Research Service, Library of Parliament. https://lop.parl.ca/staticfiles/PublicWebsite/Home/ResearchPublications/BackgroundPapers/PDF/2016-35-e.pdf

Index